T0275637

CAMBRIDGE LIBRARY COLLECTION

Books of enduring scholarly value

History of Medicine

It is sobering to realise that as recently as the year in which On the Origin of Species was published, learned opinion was that diseases such as typhus and cholera were spread by a 'miasma', and suggestions that doctors should wash their hands before examining patients were greeted with mockery by the profession. The Cambridge Library Collection reissues milestone publications in the history of Western medicine as well as studies of other medical traditions. Its coverage ranges from Galen on anatomical procedures to Florence Nightingale's common-sense advice to nurses, and includes early research into genetics and mental health, colonial reports on tropical diseases, documents on public health and military medicine, and publications on spa culture and medicinal plants.

A Treatise on Diet

The physician and author John Ayrton Paris (1785–1856), several of whose other medical and popular works have been reissued in the Cambridge Library Collection, published this book on the significance of diet to health in 1826. In the first part, Paris discusses the physiology of the digestive system, and the way that sensations of hunger, thirst and fullness are conveyed. In the second part, he considers types of food and drink, and methods of cookery. Paris suggests the times of day at which different meals should be taken, and the types and amounts of food and drink to be consumed. Part 3 deals with the problems of indigestion. A table of matters for investigation is given which covers the patient's lifestyle and habits as well as their immediate physical symptoms, and Paris firmly makes the point that changes of lifestyle are at least as important as medicine in effecting a cure.

Cambridge University Press has long been a pioneer in the reissuing of out-of-print titles from its own backlist, producing digital reprints of books that are still sought after by scholars and students but could not be reprinted economically using traditional technology. The Cambridge Library Collection extends this activity to a wider range of books which are still of importance to researchers and professionals, either for the source material they contain, or as landmarks in the history of their academic discipline.

Drawing from the world-renowned collections in the Cambridge University Library and other partner libraries, and guided by the advice of experts in each subject area, Cambridge University Press is using state-of-the-art scanning machines in its own Printing House to capture the content of each book selected for inclusion. The files are processed to give a consistently clear, crisp image, and the books finished to the high quality standard for which the Press is recognised around the world. The latest print-on-demand technology ensures that the books will remain available indefinitely, and that orders for single or multiple copies can quickly be supplied.

The Cambridge Library Collection brings back to life books of enduring scholarly value (including out-of-copyright works originally issued by other publishers) across a wide range of disciplines in the humanities and social sciences and in science and technology.

A Treatise on Diet

*With a View to Establish, on Practical Grounds,
a System of Rules, for the Prevention and Cure
of the Diseases Incident to a Disordered State
of the Digestive Functions*

JOHN AYRTON PARIS

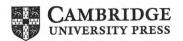

CAMBRIDGE
UNIVERSITY PRESS

CAMBRIDGE
UNIVERSITY PRESS

University Printing House, Cambridge, CB2 8BS, United Kingdom

Cambridge University Press is part of the University of Cambridge.
It furthers the University's mission by disseminating knowledge in the pursuit of
education, learning and research at the highest international levels of excellence.

www.cambridge.org
Information on this title: www.cambridge.org/9781108069892

© in this compilation Cambridge University Press 2014

This edition first published 1826
This digitally printed version 2014

ISBN 978-1-108-06989-2 Paperback

A

TREATISE

ON

DIET:

WITH A VIEW TO ESTABLISH, ON PRACTICAL GROUNDS,

A SYSTEM OF RULES,

FOR

THE PREVENTION AND CURE

OF

The Diseases

INCIDENT TO A DISORDERED STATE OF THE

DIGESTIVE FUNCTIONS.

BY

J. A. PARIS, M.D. F.R.S.

FELLOW OF THE ROYAL COLLEGE OF PHYSICIANS,

ETC. ETC.

" Some Physiologists will have it that the Stomach is a Mill; — others, that it is a
fermenting Vat; — others, again, that it is a Stew-pan; — but in my view of the
matter, it is neither a Mill, a fermenting Vat, nor a Stew-pan — but a STOMACH,
Gentlemen, a STOMACH."— *Manuscript Note from Hunter's Lectures.*

LONDON:

PRINTED FOR THOMAS & GEORGE UNDERWOOD,

32, FLEET STREET.

M.DCCC.XXVI.

CONTENTS.

PART I.

PART II.

A TREATISE ON DIET,

ETC. ETC.

INTRODUCTION.

Apology for the Work.—Popular interest of the Subject.—
Works on Dietetics, numerous, but not satisfactory.—
Contrariety of Opinion begets Scepticism.—The fate of
a Patient who consults too many Physicians.—The
quantity of Food, and the circumstances under which it
is taken, more important than its quality.—Dietetic
Precepts should not savour of ascetic austerities.—Ab-
surdity of the supposition that Nature can direct us in
the selection of Food.—Man has no natural Food.—
The qualities of Vegetables completely changed by Cul-
tivation.—Cookery.—The folly of denying the influence
of Regimen in the cure and prevention of Disease.—
Digestion, comprehensive Signification of the Term.

IN these days of literary fecundity, an author who ventures to add a new work upon a subject which has already
given birth to so many volumes, must be able to satisfy
the public tribunal, that he is either prepared to extend
the general stock of information, or to correct the errors
into which preceding writers have been betrayed. I shall
certainly, upon the present occasion, rely with greater confidence upon this latter plan of defence. It will be readily
admitted that few subjects, connected with the medical art,

B

have excited more popular interest, or occasioned more sedulous inquiry, than that of which I propose to treat in the following pages ; and yet, were the numerous works on dietetics subjected to a healthy digestion, how meagre would be the proportion of real aliment extracted from their bulky materials. Upon this occasion, at least, we may, with Diderot, ridicule the popular adage, " *the more heads the better counsel—because nothing is more common than heads, and nothing so unusual as good advice.*" Suppose an unprejudiced reader, my assumption I admit is violent, were to wade through the discordant mass to which I allude, would he not inevitably arrive at the mortifying conclusion, that nothing is known upon the subject in question ; or rather, that there does not exist any necessity for such knowledge ? Nothing cherishes the public scepticism, with regard to the efficacy of the medical art, so much, as the publication of the adverse and contradictory opinions of its professors, upon points so apparently simple and obvious, that every superficially informed person constitutes himself a judge of their merits. If a reader is informed by one class of authors, that a weak stomach is unable to convert *liquid* food into aliment, and by another, that *solid* food is injurious to feeble stomachs, he at once infers that the question is one of perfect indifference ; and he ultimately arrives, by a very simple process of reasoning, at the sweeping conclusion, that the stomach, ever kind and accommodating, indiscriminately converts every species of food into nourishment, and that he has therefore only to consult his own inclination in its selection. On the valetudinarian, incapable of healthy reflection, and ever seeking for causes of fear and anxiety when they do not choose to come uncalled, such works may have a contrary tendency, and lead him to suspect the seeds of disease in every dish, and poison in every cup.

2. To make the case still stronger, let us suppose that the unprejudiced person, whom we have chosen to repre-

sent on this occasion, instead of a reader becomes a patient, and submits his complaints to the judgment of these discordant authors; might he not, like the Emperor Adrian, prepare an inscription * for his tomb-stone? This is not an imaginary case, but one of daily occurrence in this metropolis. A dyspeptic invalid, restless and impatient from the nature of his complaints, wanders from physician to physician, and from surgeon to surgeon, in the eager expectation of procuring some relief from his sufferings: under the direction of one, he takes the blue pill, and, like Sanctorius, measures with scrupulous accuracy the prescribed quantity of his ingesta; but, disappointed in the promised benefit, he solicits other advice, and is mortified by hearing that mercury, in every form of combination, must aggravate the evils he seeks to cure, and that a generous diet, and bitter stomachics, are alone calculated to meet the exigencies of his case; a trial is given to the plan, but with no better success: the unhappy patient at length determines to leave his case to nature; but at this critical juncture he meets a sympathizing friend, by whom he is earnestly entreated to apply to a skilful physician, who had succeeded in curing a similar complaint, under which he had himself severely laboured: the anxious sufferer, with renewed confidence, sends for this long sought for doctor, and he hears, with a mixture of horror and astonishment, that his disorder has been entirely mistaken, and that he must submit to the mortifications of a hermit, or his cure is hopeless. It is unnecessary to pursue the history; but I appeal to the candid and enlightened members of the profession to say, whether I have caricatured the portrait. No one can believe that I intend to cast the slightest reproach upon any practitioner by these observations; it is to the unsettled state of professional opinion upon the subject of diet, and to the obscurity which involves the

---

* " It was the *great number* of physicians that killed the Emperor."

theory of digestion, that all these evils are to be solely attributed. But to return to the subject of dietetic works; it appears to me that their authors have laid far too great stress upon the quality of the different species of food, and have condemned particular aliments for those effects which should be attributed to the quantity, and circumstances under which they were taken; their dietetic precepts have frequently assumed the air of ascetic austerities, and they have thus represented the cure far more formidable than the disease. It has been sarcastically observed by a popular writer, more remarkable for the playfulness of his style than the soundness of his arguments, that there exists a more intimate connexion between the doctrine of Tertullian and that of many a dietetic practitioner, than is generally supposed — that he is the ascetic intrenched in gallipots and blisters, preaching against beef and porter; terrifying his audience with fire and brimstone in one age, and in the other, with gout and apoplexy. Now, while we must all deeply lament that the severity of this sarcasm should have been, in some measure, sanctioned by the theoretical absurdities of many of our minor writers, it is impossible that any reasonable person can seriously contend, that numerous diseases do not arise from an improper management of diet; much less, that a judicious regulation of it cannot be rendered subservient to their cure.

3. It has been affirmed with an air of much confidence, that the management of our diet requires not the aid of reason or philosophy, since Nature has implanted in us instincts sufficiently strong and intelligible to direct us to what is salutary, and to warn us from such aliments as are injurious. We may here observe, that man has so long forsaken the simple laws which Nature had instituted for his direction, that it is to be feared she has abandoned her charge, and left him under the control of that faithless guide and usurper, to which civilisation has given dominion. Appetite, which expresses the true wants of the

system, can no longer be distinguished from that feeling which induces us to prefer one species of food to another, and which entirely depends on habit, and certain associations. That the natural relations which subsist between the qualities of food and the impressions made by them on the senses, are changed or destroyed by the refinements of artificial life, is a fact supported by too many powerful arguments to refute : how many kinds of aliments, originally disagreeable, become pleasant by habit; and how many substances, naturally agreeable, become disgusting from the creation of certain prejudices ! I am acquainted with a lady who is constantly made sick by eating a green oyster; the cause of which may be traced to an erroneous impression she received with respect to the nature of the colouring matter being cupreous. It has also been frequently observed, that persons in social life have acquired a preternatural sensibility to vegetable odours, while the savage has a keener sense for the exhalations of animal bodies: we are, for instance, assured by Captain Cook, that the people of Kamschatka did not smell a vegetable essence placed near them, but that they discovered, by their olfactory sense, a rotten fish, or a stranded whale, at a considerable distance.

4. Dr. George Fordyce has urged a still more serious and conclusive objection to that hackneyed maxim—" that we ought to live *naturally*, and on such food as is presented to us by nature;" viz. that *man has no natural food.* It is decreed that he shall earn his bread by the sweat of his brow ; or in other words, that he shall, by his industry, discover substances from whence he is to procure subsistence.; and that if he cannot find such, he must cultivate and alter them from their natural state. There is scarcely a vegetable which we at present employ, that can be found growing naturally : Buffon states, that our wheat is a factitious production, raised to its present condition by the

art of agriculture. Rice, rye, barley, or even oats, are not
to be found wild; that is to say, growing naturally in any
part of the earth, but have been altered, by the industry
of mankind, from plants not now resembling them even in
such a degree as to enable us to recognise their relations.
The acrid and disagreeable *apium graveolens* has been thus
transformed into delicious celery ; and the *colewort*, a plant
of scanty leaves, not weighing altogether half an ounce,
has been improved into cabbage, whose leaves alone weigh
many pounds, or into a cauliflower of considerable dimensions, being only the embryo of a few buds, which, in their
natural state, would not have weighed many grains. The
potatoe, again, whose introduction has added many mil-
lions to our population, derives its origin from a small and
bitter root, which grows wild in Chili and at Monte
Video.* These few instances may suffice to answer the
object for which they were introduced : the reader will
find many others in the Introduction to my Pharmacologia.†

5. If cultivation can ever be said to have left the trans-
formation of vegetables imperfect, the genius of cookery is
certainly entitled to the merit of having completed it ; for,
whatever traces of natural qualities may have remained,
they are undoubtedly obliterated during their passage
through her potent alembic. It has been observed, that
the useful object of cookery is to render aliments agreeable
to the senses, and of easy digestion ; in short, to spare the
stomach a drudgery which can be more easily performed
by a spit or stewpan, — that of loosening the texture, or
softening the fibres of the food; and which are essential
preliminaries to its digestion. A no less important effect
is produced by rendering it more palatable; for it is a fact,
which I shall have to consider on a future occasion, that

* See Pharmacologia, edit. 6. vol. i. p. 147.   † Ibid. p. 114.

the gratification which attends a favourite meal is, in itself, a specific stimulus to the organs of digestion, especially in weak and debilitated habits.

6. Experience can alone supply the want of instinct; and, unless we assume this as the basis of all our inquiries upon the subject of diet, our theories, however refined, and supported by chemical and physiological researches, will prove but Will-o'-th'-wisps, to lead us astray into numerous difficulties and embarrassments. Experience, for instance, dearly bought experience, has taught us that headach, flatulency, hypochondriasis, and a thousand nameless ills, have arisen from the too prevailing fashion of loading our tables with that host of French *entremets,* and *hors-d'œuvres,* which have so unfortunately usurped the roast beef of old England. The theorists, in the true spirit of philosophical refinement, laugh at our terrors; they admit, to be sure, that the man who eats round the table, " *ab ovo usque ad mala,*" is a terrific glutton, but that, after all, *he has only eaten words;* for, eat as he may, he can only eat animal matter, vegetable matter, and condiment, either cooked by the heat of water or by that of fire, figure or disfigure, serve, arrange, flavour, or adorn them as you please. There is no physician of any practical knowledge who cannot, at once, refute such a doctrine; every nurse knows, from experience, that certain mixtures produce deleterious compounds in the stomach, although the chemist may perhaps fail in explaining their nature, or the theory of their formation. What would such a reasoner say, if he were invited to a repast, and were presented only with charcoal and water? would he be reconciled to his fare by being told that his discontent was founded on a mere delusion? that the difference between them and the richest vegetable viands was merely ideal, an affair of words, as in either case he would only swallow *oxygen, hydrogen,* and carbon? and yet the presumption in such a case would not be more violent, nor would the

argument be less tenable, than that by which the chemist attempts to defend the innocence of a practice which converts our refreshments into burdens, and our food into poison. To those who question the value of dietetic regulations in the cure of disease, I have only to observe, that they may as well deny the utility of the medical art altogether, and assert that in all disorders of function, Nature is sufficiently powerful to rectify and cure them, without the intervention of art : unless this be granted, it is absurd to say that beneficial impressions may not be made as well through the medium of the *materia alimentaria,* as through that of the *materia medica ;* or, to borrow the language of Dr. Arbuthnot, that what we take daily by POUNDS must be, at least, as important as what we take seldom, and only by grains or tea-spoonsful.

7. Those who have read my work on Pharmacology, will easily discover the train of research by which my mind has been led, from the study of the operation of medicines, to that of the digestion of aliment; while those who are acquainted with the various works on dietetics will readily admit, that an ample apology may be found for giving to the public another volume on that subject. Upon this point, however, I wish to be distinctly understood; for I should be seriously concerned at being identified with a school, which uniformly depresses the opinions and writings of others, in order that those of their own immediate disciples may rise in relative importance. It would be worse than foolish to assert that, upon the subject of dietetics, we have no works of merit; the valuable treatise of Dr. Fordyce would, singly, be sufficient to repel with triumph a charge so illiberal and unjust : at the same time, it cannot be denied, that since the periods in which many excellent works were composed, physiology, as well as chemistry, has advanced with rapid strides ; pathology has thrown off the mystic veil with which the humoral doctrine had invested her, and the

views, as well as the language of medical science, have undergone corresponding revolutions. Facts alone remain unchanged ; but those are so buried in the ruins of the fallen fabric, that, unless they be rescued from the confused mass, their intrinsic value must be entirely lost : any work, therefore, carefully collated, with the view of accomplishing such an object, even should it present but little novelty, must prove an acceptable offering to the intelligent part of the community.

8. Before the subject of dietetics can be systematically considered, or the principles upon which disease may be prevented or cured by an appropriate diet, can be properly understood, or profitably applied, the reader must be made acquainted with the complicated machinery by which Nature extracts blood from food. The various processes engaged in this wonderful transmutation are expressed by the comprehensive term DIGESTION, although this word is sometimes employed in a more limited sense, to denote only those preparatory changes which the food undergoes in the stomach. Mr. Abernethy would appear to use the term according to this latter acceptation, for he says,—" *Digestion* takes place in the stomach, *chylification* in the small intestines, and a third process, hitherto undenominated, is performed in the large intestines." The relation of a tale which has been so often told, may, perhaps, appear to many as not only superfluous but reprehensible; I must, however, remark, that every author is conventionally allowed to state the theme of his discussion in his own language, and the advantages which have hitherto attended the indulgence sufficiently sanction its continuance.

ANATOMICAL VIEW OF THE DIGESTIVE ORGANS.

Their elaborate Machinery.—Their Structure varies according to the Food of the Animal to which they belong. — Enumeration of the several digestive Organs. — Their extraordinary sympathetic relations.—The ALIMENTARY CANAL :—*its peristaltic Motion.—The Stomach :—its Figure, Dimensions, Situation, and Structure. — Small Intestines. — The Duodenum : — Peculiarities of its Functions entitle it to be considered as a second Stomach :—Provisions to limit its Motions.— Jejunum.—Ilium.—Large Intestines.—Cæcum.—Colon. — Rectum. — The* VARIOUS GLANDS, OR SECRETING ORGANS, FOR THE PREPARATION OF THE DIGESTIVE FLUIDS.—*The salivary Glands.—Glands of the Stomach and Intestines.—The Liver.—The Pancreas.— Observations on the supposed Use of the Spleen.* —VESSELS FOR CARRYING THE NUTRITIVE PRODUCT TO THE CURRENT OF THE CIRCULATION.— *The Lacteals. — Mesenteric Glands. — The Thoracic Duct.—The* LUNGS.—*The* KIDNEYS.—*The* SKIN.

9. No function in the animal economy presents such elaborate machinery as that of digestion; but its complexity and extent have been found to vary according to the nature of the food upon which it is designed to act. If it greatly differ in composition from the matter of which the animal is constituted, the changes it has to undergo before it can be adapted for the support and reparation of the body which receives it, must necessarily be more considerable, and the organs are accordingly more extensive and elaborate in herbivorous than in carnivorous animals; while man, who derives his supplies of nourish-

ment from both the kingdoms of nature, possesses an intermediate organization. His digestive organs may be said
to consist of a long canal, extending from the mouth to
the anus, varying in the diameter of its different parts,
according to the distinct duties which each is destined to
perform; and which are also capable of contracting or
enlarging their dimensions according to the circumstances
under which they act;—of various glands, or secreting
organs, for the preparation of the liquids which are required for acting on the alimentary matters; — of vessels
for conveying to the current of the circulation the nutritive
product of the operation; — of the lungs, which complete
its assimilation with the blood; — and of the kidneys,
which carry off the remaining portion as excrementitious.
These different organs are not only intimately connected
with each other, but they display an extraordinary sympathetic relation with the sanguiferous and cerebral systems : there is, for instance, no organ of the body which
is not directly or indirectly affected by the operations of
the stomach : we shall therefore cease to wonder that an
impression made upon it by a medicinal agent, or by an
alimentary substance, should afford the means of exciting
an action in the most distant parts of the machine; nor
can we be surprised that the aberrations of this central
organ should give origin to the greater number of maladies
with which the body is afflicted ; or, that those applications
should be so effective which are directed, for their cure,
through the medium of its sympathies.   But that we may
not, like the members in the ancient fable, wage an
unjust war against the stomach for the maladies which
it may thus inflict, it is necessary to state, that the stomach
suffers equally, in its turn, from the derangement of
distant organs.   What practitioner has not witnessed the
sudden sickness produced by the sprains of tendinous and
ligamentous structures, or by blows on the head or other
parts? To distinguish between the sympathetic and pri-

mary affections of the digestive organs, is a problem of
the greatest practical importance; and the profession is
much indebted to Mr. Abernethy for his endeavours to
shew how the stomach and bowels may become affected
from local disorder.

10. Although it would be obviously foreign to the
plan and objects of this work to enter into minute anatomical investigations, yet as there are certain facts, connected with the structure and locality of the alimentary
organs, which it is essential for the practitioner to bear in
mind, I shall here offer such a description of them as may
appear necessary for his guidance, or for the maintenance
of that perspicuity which I am anxious to bestow upon
the following pages. In the performance of this task, I
shall preserve the order of arrangement already noticed (9),
viz.—

I. The Alimentary Canal.

11. Although, in strict language, the alimentary canal
includes the whole passage from the mouth to the anus,
the term is more usually employed to express only the
stomach and intestinal tube. It may be represented as a
long canal, commonly calculated as being five or six times
the length of the adult, differently twisted upon itself,
and of different dimensions in various parts of its extent.
Anatomists describe it as composed of several distinct
tunics, or coats, the existence of which may be traced
throughout its whole extent, although their structure
undergoes variation in the different divisions of the canal;
but this will be better understood when we come to speak
of its individual parts. The intestinal canal is susceptible
of a peculiar motion, which arises from the successive
or simultaneous contraction of its longitudinal or circular
fibres, and has been differently denominated by authors;
some have named it *vermicular*, others *peristaltic*. This

contraction always takes place slowly, and in an irregular manner; it is, however, capable of being accelerated by the action of certain stimulants. It does not seem to be sensibly controlled by the will; nor, indeed, does it appear to be much influenced by the nervous system, for it proceeds in the stomach after the section of the eighth pair of nerves, and it even continues, though the intestinal canal be entirely separated from the body : at the same time it appears, from the experiments related by Dr. W. Phillip, that, although these muscular fibres be independent of the nervous system, they may in every instance be influenced through it; a fact of very great pathological importance, since it follows that the muscular fibres of the canal may not only be affected by causes acting directly on them, but by such as act through the medium of their nerves. M. Majendie observes, that the peristaltic motion becomes more active by the weakness of animals, and even by their death; and that in some, by this cause, it becomes considerably accelerated. The object of this motion is to propel forward the contents of the canal, and to favour those changes which it is destined to undergo. The intestinal canal is never in a state of complete collapse, it always contains gas or vapour, which prevents its sides from coming into contact. It has been stated that this canal is of different dimensions in various parts of its extent, and it is principally from this diversity of magnitude that anatomists have established those divisions which we have next to consider.

12. The stomach is a membranous bag, very much resembling in shape that of the pouch of a bag-pipe, or, more strictly speaking, that of a conoid bent upon itself. It is not easy to determine its exact capacity in the living body, nor is it a fact of much practical importance : in various states of disease, we have reason to believe that it is considerably augmented in size. It has two orifices ; the one termed the *cardia*, which is a termination of the

tube we call the œsophagus; the other, which communicates with the small intestine, and to which the term
pylorus has been given. The pylorus is raised up, being
nearly, but not quite level with the cardia, so that its
upper and lower surfaces form, as it were, two concentric
circles, one on the upper side, which is called the small
curvature, and one on the lower, which is termed the great
curvature. The stomach is situated immediately below
the diaphragm, the *cardia* being nearly opposite to the
middle of the vertebræ. From thence it bulges out to the
left side, the great curvature coming forward and down-
ward; it then passes on to the right side, rising upwards,
so that the *pylorus* is not much farther from the diaphragm than the *cardia;* when, therefore, a man is in an
erect posture, substances must ascend to pass through the
pylorus. It is, however, evident that its situation, and
relation with the neighbouring organs, will always suffer
variations according to its degree of distention; the following observations will therefore deserve the attention of
the pathologist : — in its flaccid state, it occupies the
epigastrium and part of the left *hypochondrium;* whilst,
when distended, it exchanges its flattened, for a rounded
form, and fills almost completely the left *hypochondrium;*
the greater curvature descends towards the umbilicus,
particularly on the left side : on account of the resistance
that the vertebral column presents, the posterior surface
of the stomach cannot distend itself in that direction;
this viscus is therefore wholly carried forward. This
dilatation of the stomach produces very important changes
in the abdomen: the total volume of the cavity aug-
ments; the belly juts out; the abdominal viscera are
compressed with greater force; and the necessity of passing
urine or fæces is frequently experienced. At the same
time, the diaphragm is pressed towards the breast, and it
descends with some difficulty; whence the respiratory
motions are impeded. The stomach, although a single

bag, must be considered as divisible into two distinct
cavities, to which different offices are evidently assigned.
The left half has always larger dimensions than the right;
and M. Majendie calls the one the *splenic* part, because it
is supported on the spleen, and the other the *pyloric* part,
since it is supported on the pylorus.

13. The stomach has been described as composed of
several membranes, viz., the *peritonæal, muscular, nervous,*
and *villous* coats. The nervous coat, however, of Haller
and the old anatomists, is now acknowledged to be nothing
more than cellular membrane; and we might with equal
propriety dismiss the two former from the number. The
peritonæal covering, being common to all the contents of
the abdomen, can scarcely be recognised as one of the
proper coats of the stomach; while it has been very justly
observed, that the muscular fibres, arranged between the
peritonæum and the villous membrane, cannot maintain
the name of a *coat* with propriety, since the term signifies
a containing membrane, whereas the muscular fibres owe
their connection with each other to interposed cellular
membrane. There remains, then, only the villous membrane; and this, in fact, is the only proper intestinal
coat, or containing membrane of the aliment. The same
observations will apply to the structure of the alimentary
canal generally.

14. The villous, or mucous membrane, has a whitish-
red appearance, and presents a singular velvet-like appearance, from which it has derived its name; not being
elastic, it has numerous folds, or *rugæ*, which supply this
deficiency, and serve to accommodate the capacity of the
stomach to the bulk of its contents; and, at the same
time, to retain the aliment until it is duly elaborated. It
is usually lined with a mucous matter, especially in its
splenic extremity; it also contains many follicles; and
near the pylorus are to be seen several glands, to which is
assigned a peculiar office, to be hereafter described. The

stomach is abundantly vascular; indeed it may be observed that few structures receive so much blood as this organ; four arteries, three of which are considerable, are exclusively devoted to its service; and their several branches communicate most freely with each other in all directions, by innumerable anastomoses; and, being tortuous, they can thus accommodate themselves to the full and empty states of the cavity. Nor are its nerves less numerous; they are composed of the eighth pair, and a great many filaments proceeding from the *solar plexus* of the great *sympathetic*. At the pylorus the mucous membrane thickens, and forms a circular fold, which performs the office of a valve; a fibrous dense tissue is also here found, which some authors have called the *pyloric muscle*.

15. *The duodenum* comprehends that range of small intestine which commences at the pylorus, and extends for about twelve inches; and so important are the changes which the aliment undergoes in its cavity, that many authors have regarded it as entitled to the appellation of a second stomach; and I shall, hereafter, have occasion to state, that many diseases which have been erroneously attributed to the stomach, derive their origin from the functional aberrations of this intestine; a fact which renders a knowledge of its structure and situation of great importance to the pathologist. Unlike the stomach, which may be said to be comparatively loose and floating in the abdominal cavity, it is secured in its position by various attachments, and the manner it is protected strongly evinces the importance of its functions. The practitioner should ever keep in mind the position and bearings of this intestine; for, as Dr. Yeats has justly observed, and the fact has been confirmed by my own experience, that patients, directed by their own uneasy feelings, will frequently trace, with most anatomical accuracy, the course of the duodenum with their finger, from the stomach to the loins on the right side, and back again across the abdomen to the umbilicus.

The duodenum, at its commencement, turns backwards and downwards for a short way; it then turns towards the right kidney, to the capsule of which it is more or less attached; it here forms a sacculated angle, and in this depending part, the ducts for conveying the pancreatic and biliary secretions enter the intestine; it now ascends from the right to the left, just before the aorta and the last vertebræ of the back; it continues this direction from thence obliquely forward by a slight curvature, and makes its exit through the ring in the mesentery. Its mucous membrane, which presents many villi, and a great number of follicles for the secretion of its own peculiar fluid, forms irregular circular folds, termed " *Valvulæ Conniventes,*" which increase the surface of the intestine, while they prevent the too rapid passage of its contents. It is furnished with nerves from the *ganglions of the great sympathetic;* and it is also abundantly supplied with bloodvessels. It is impossible to view all the arrangements of this organ, without being satisfied that Nature was anxious to limit its motions; and a little reflection will convince us of the great importance of such a provision: Dr. Yeats, in his valuable paper on the duodenum,[*] which is published in the sixth volume of the Transactions of the College, has alluded to this fact in a very pointed manner. It is evident that, had this intestine been loose and floating, the food might have passed too rapidly through it; it might also have drawn the small end of the stomach out of its proper situation; and there would have been a constant disposition in the food to pass out of the stomach into the duodenum, upon every relaxation of the pylorus: besides which, had it been less confined, and consequently subject to greater distension, a regurgitation

---

[*] Some Observations on the Duodenum; with plates descriptive of its situation and connexions. Extracted from the Gulstonian Lectures, by G. D. Yeats, M.D., &c.

might have taken place into the *ductus communis,* from an alteration in that obliquity of its direction, which now so securely guards against such an occurrence. Dr. Fordyce, in noticing the fact of the peritonæum being wanting on the back of the duodenum, most erroneously concludes that this was ordained with a view of allowing a greater distension than can take place in the lower intestines; had such been the design of Nature, she certainly would not have discarded so highly elastic a membrane, and attached the back of the duodenum to the vertebræ.

16. The *Jejunum.* The precise point at which the duodenum terminates, and the jejunum commences, cannot perhaps be accurately defined; but this latter intestine is generally considered as beginning where the mesentery takes its rise. It appears to have derived its name from the fact of its usually being found empty; probably from its more rapid powers of absorption.

17. The *Ilium* is the continuation of the jejunum, and is the last division of the small intestine; it is said to have derived its name from the manner in which it is coiled up by the mesentery. Its parietes are thinner than those of the preceding portion of the canal, and this circumstance, together with the deep yellow colour of its contents, impart to it an appearance very distinct from that of the duodenum.

18. The large intestines exceed the others in diameter, but are less considerable in length; in structure they also differ considerably from the small intestines; their mucous membrane does not present that villous appearance of which we have spoken; but is, on the contrary, smooth: the number of follicles is also less, and it is supplied with much fewer arteries, veins, and nerves.

19. The *Cæcum* constitutes the first division of this portion of the intestinal canal, although some anatomists consider it as merely the head of the colon, and restrict the term *cæcum* to a small gut which is usually described under the

title of *Appendix Vermiformis,* and which takes its rise from the posterior part of the cæcum ; it is about the size of a quill, resembling, in figure and diameter, a common earth worm : its coats contain numerous mucous glands, and its cavity, which communicates freely with that of the cæcum, is usually filled with a thick mucous fluid : its use is not well understood, but it is evidently designed to supply a fluid of some kind ; and as the essential parts of the digestion are completed before the aliment arrives at this part, we may fairly conclude that the object of such fluid is to lubricate the intestinal passage, and thus to facilitate the expulsion of the fæces. At its junction with the ilium, the cæcum, or, according to some anatomists, the colon, exhibits a valve, formed by the production of the interior coat of the intestine, evidently disposed to permit matters to pass forwards, but to prevent their return into the ilium.

20. The *Colon* constitutes the principal tract of the large intestines, and exceeds them all in diameter : as accumulations in its cavity frequently produce various ill effects from their pressure, it becomes essential for the practitioner to know its direction and bearings. It commences in the cavity of the os ilium, on the right side ; from thence, ascending by the kidney on the same side, it passes under the concave side of the liver, to which it is sometimes tied, as also to the gall bladder, which tinges it yellow in that place;* it then runs under the bottom of the stomach to the spleen, in the left side, to which it is also affixed ; and thence, passing in the form of the Greek letter Σ, it terminates in the upper part of the os sacrum in the rectum. It appears, therefore, to be contiguous to all the digestive organs, and may consequently produce much disturbance by its morbid disten-

---

* At least such is its appearance in the dead subject ; whether a similar transudation takes place during life, is very doubtful.

sion ; its connexion with the duodenum is also a circumstance of much pathological importance : whatever motion
takes place in the former intestine, will be communicated,
more or less, to the latter ; and should it become unnaturally distended, it will press immediately upon the ascending part of the duodenum, and retard the progress of the
alimentary matter, which has always to rise against gravity,
when the body is in an erect position, or recumbent on
the right side.   The colon has been divided into the
ascending portion, which extends from the cæcum to the
right hypochondrium ; into the *transverse* portion, or what
is termed its *great arch ;* and into the descending portion,
including what has been called its *sigmoid flexure.*   The
coats of this intestine are much stronger than those of the
others ; its muscular layer has also a peculiar disposition ;
its longitudinal fibres form three straight bundles or bands,
far separated from each other when the intestine is dilated ;
at the same time, its circular fibres form bands, equally
separated from each other, but more numerous : from
which arrangement, it follows, that in a great number of
places, the intestine only consists of the peritonæum and
its mucous membrane ; these places are generally formed
into distinct cavities, which have been termed the *cells
of the colon ;* they serve to promote a gradual descent of
the excrement ; but, when the action of the canal is
torpid, they give origin to much mischief, by unduly
retaining its contents.

21. Several physiologists have supposed that the colon
performs some other function than that of a mere recipient.
Sir E. Home imagined that it formed fat ; an hypothesis
which would have received some slight support from the
fact that the fattest animals have generally the largest
colons, did we not know that persons have lived, and
enjoyed good health, for many years, with an artificial
anus formed by the cecal extremity of the small intestines,
which sufficiently proves that the large intestines are

not essential to perfect digestion, nor to the maintenance of life.

22. The *Rectum* is the last portion of the intestinal canal; it begins at the upper part of the os sacrum, where the colon ends, and going straight down (whence its name), it is tied to the extremities of the coccyx by the peritonæum behind, and to the neck of the bladder in men, but in women to the vagina uteri before; whence arises the sympathy between those parts. The coats of the rectum are more thick and fleshy than those of any other of the intestines: it has in general no valves, but several rugæ; had the former existed, the expulsion of the fæces would have suffered inconvenient delay. The figure of the rectum varies, as it is full or empty; when empty, it is regularly cylindrical, and contracts in transverse folds: it is capable of very great distension, and may even be extended to the size of a large bladder: the quantity of fæces that sometimes accumulates is prodigious, and cannot be removed except by mechanical means.

II. *The various Glands which are subservient to the Secretion of the different Fluids intended to act on the Alimentary Matter.*

23. There is nothing more mysterious in the digestive process than the great variety of the different fluids which appear essential for its completion; each of which has appropriate glands for its secretion. These fluids are, the *saliva,* which is formed by glands whose secretory ducts open into the mouth; and *mucous matter,* which results from the action of numerous follicles situated in the interior of the cheeks and palate, upon the back of the tongue, on the anterior aspect of the *velum* and on the *uvula;*—the *gastric juice,* formed by glands in the stomach; and the

mucus secreted by its membrane ;—the " *succus intestinalis,*"
or proper juice of the duodenum and small intestines ; —
the *bile,* which being secreted in the liver, and rendered
more stimulating in the gall-bladder, is afterwards carried
into the duodenum ;—the *pancreatic juice,* which is secreted
in the pancreas, and carried into the duodenum along with
the bile ; to which may, perhaps, be added the *watery
liquids* thrown into the intestines by the exhalants.   Were
I to describe the intimate structure of the several glands
and vessels which furnish these fluids, we should be led
into anatomical details of tedious length, and which would
be wholly unattended by practical utility.   It is, however,
essential for the physiologist, as well as the practitioner,
to become acquainted with the most recent account of the
chemical history of these several secreted fluids.

24. The *Saliva.* The mixture under this name is probably variable in its physical and chemical properties,
according to circumstances which have not hitherto been
examined.   When first discharged from the mouth, it
always holds suspended a *mucus,* which is not dissolved,
but imparts to it a frothy quality, by enabling it to retain
the air which it absorbs from the atmosphere.   It is
readily separated by merely diluting the saliva as it flows
from the mouth, with distilled water, when it will gradually
subside, and may be collected on a filter.   It is a curious
circumstance that, although no traces of *phosphate of lime*
can be detected in this mucus by the application of
reagents, yet, after incineration, a considerable proportion
appears in the ash.*   It has been doubted whether this
mucus be secreted by the salivary glands, or is the
common mucus of the mouth ; the latter appears more

* It is this mucus that produces the *tartar* of the teeth, which, at first,
is only mucus precipitated on the surface of the enamel ; but it soon
begins to decompose ; its colour changes, by the influence of the air, from
white to yellow ; the warmth and moisture of the mouth contribute to
complete the decomposition, and the same earthy phosphates, which are

probable. The saliva, deprived of this mucus, consists, according to the analysis by Berzetius, of

Water.......................	992·9
A peculiar animal matter	2·9
Alkaline muriates	1·7
Lactate of soda and animal matter	0·9
Pure soda	9

The peculiar matter of the saliva is soluble in water, but not in alcohol; and the solution is not precipitated either by alkalies or acids, or sub-acetate of lead, or muriate of mercury, or tannin; neither is it rendered turbid by boiling. The saliva derives its name from the saline qualities which it possesses; and although, under ordinary circumstances, we are not conscious of them, yet when the stomach has been long empty, and the nervous system acquires increased sensibility, the saline taste is frequently perceptible. The same effect is produced by disease; and the disagreeable taste of which invalids complain, often depends upon chemical changes having been produced in this secreted fluid. The common furred tongue would appear to arise from an increased quantity of vitiated mucus. The peculiar milky tongue * which appears in certain states of the system, occasionally derives its appearance from an innumerable number of microscopic bubbles of air, as I have ascertained by observation: in such cases, the quantity, rather than the quality of the mucus, appears to be affected. The black tongue of typhus, on the other hand, is indebted for its character to a decomposed state of the mucus; while a deficiency in

---

produced by oxidation and combustion in open fire, are here formed, and slowly deposited on the surface of the tooth by a slower but a similar process. The *tartar* is therefore, as it were, the *ash* of mucus crystallized on the tooth.

* I am induced to consider the milky tongue as rather indicating a *sympathetic*, than *primary* derangement of the stomach. It is thus constantly produced by mental anxiety.

the true salivary secretion will explain its dryness. It must at the same time be confessed, that there are certain morbid conditions of the tongue which cannot be explained upon these principles, much less can we discover the nature of their connexion with those diseases which are known to produce them. I am, for instance, at a loss to understand why the tongue should be clean in certain stages of hectic fever, at the very time that the stomach is palpably deranged : and thus again, although experience has established the fact, how are we to explain why an unnaturally red tongue, of a cherry colour, when accompanied with tenderness in the epigastric region, should denote organic mischief in the alimentary organs ? I am so perfectly satisfied of the truth of this statement, from experience, that if a patient applies to me with aggravated symptoms of dyspepsia, and I perceive his tongue to be bright, I form an unfavourable diagnosis of his case. I state this as a general proposition, to which of course there will be many exceptions.

When we consider the size of the salivary glands, which altogether cannot weigh more than four ounces, the quantity of fluid which they continually secrete is truly astonishing. It would be a difficult matter to ascertain, with accuracy, the proportion of saliva which these glands can separate in a given time; but we know, that a person unaccustomed to smoking, will discharge half a pint in a very short period. In the case of a felon, who cut his throat in prison, and so completely divided both the larynx, a little above the cricoid cartilage, and the œsophagus at the same point, that whatever was introduced into the mouth escaped by the external wound; it was found that, during each meal, there was a discharge of saliva from the mouth, amounting to from five or six, to eight ounces, or even more. This is sufficient to disprove the opinion of Dr. Fordyce, who says, " as far as I can judge, the secretion during a meal can hardly exceed an ounce or two; and I should think that it serves only to lubricate the passages through which the food is to pass." With respect to this latter assumption, I shall have to offer some observations in a future part of the work.

25. The *Gastric Juice.* Great difference of opinion has existed with regard to the qualities and composition of this fluid; it would, however, appear that other secretions of a mucous nature take place in the stomach, with which it may be mixed: this circumstance, together with the difficulty of obtaining it in an isolated form, are suffi-cient to explain the contradictory results which different chemists have obtained. It is, moreover, by no means improbable that this liquor may vary in different stomachs, or even in the same stomach under different circumstances. M. Majendie observes, that the contact of different sorts of food upon the mucous membrane, may possibly influence its composition: it is, at least, certain that the gastric juice varies in different animals; for example, that of man is incapable of acting on bones, while that of the dog digests these substances perfectly. From the best autho-rities upon this subject, the true gastric juice would seem to be a glairy fluid, not very diffusible in water, and pos-sessing the power of coagulating certain fluids in a very eminent degree. Dr. Fordyce states, that six or seven grains of the inner coat of the stomach, infused in water, gave a liquor which coagulated more than a hundred ounces of milk. Some authors have regarded it as colourless, and without taste or smell, while others have described it as being acidulous.* Dr. Young, of Edinburgh, is stated to have found that an infusion of the inner coat of the stomach, which had been previously washed with water, and afterwards with a dilute solution of sub-

---

* Dr. Prout has lately read a paper before the Royal Society, in order to prove that the stomach always contains *muriatic acid.* I shall have occasion to advert to this fact in a subsequent part of the work.

carbonate of potass, still retained the power of coagulating milk very readily. We see, therefore, how unfounded that opinion is which attributes to the potation of water, the mischief of diluting the gastric fluid, and thus of weakening the digestive process. The coagulating and efficient principle, whatever it may be, is evidently not diffusible in that liquid. After one fit of vomiting, should another take place after a short interval, the matter brought up will be little more than water, with a slight saline impregnation, and some mucus; it will not be found to possess any power of coagulation; which, Dr. Fordyce observes, evidently shews that even water flowing from the exhalants, and which we should therefore expect would throw off the whole of any substance from the surface of the stomach, is incapable of detaching the gastric juice.

26. The mucous membrane of the small intestines secretes also a peculiar liquid, to which Haller gave the name of *intestinal juice;* the quantity that is formed in twenty-four hours, he estimated at eight pounds: and M. Majendie states, that if this mucous membrane be laid bare in a dog, and the layer of mucus absorbed by a sponge, it is renewed in a minute; and he says, that this observation may be repeated as often as we please, until the intestine becomes inflamed by the contact of the air, and foreign bodies. It has never been submitted to an accurate analysis; it appears, however, to be viscous, thready, of a salt taste, and capable of reddening paper tinged with turnsol.

27. The *Liver* is, by far, the largest gland in the human body, and is so disproportionate to the quantity of liquid secreted, that the bile must require a very extensive apparatus for its elaboration; and this inference is strengthened by an examination of its composition, for few fluids are so complex, and so different from the blood. A knowledge of the locality of the liver is a fact of considerable importance to the practitioner, as he is frequently called

upon to investigate diseases which depend, or are supposed to depend, upon organic changes in the structure of
this viscus. Under such circumstances, the patient must
submit to a manual examination; and the medical student who is unacquainted with the situation of the liver,
with respect to the general cavity of the abdomen, or
with the changes which its position may undergo from
various circumstances, will frequently find himself involved
in difficulty and confusion.

28. The liver is situated in the superior part of the
abdomen, principally on the right side; it generally occupies the epigastric and the right hypochondric regions;
but, since the inferior part of the chest may be diminished
in capacity, or altered in figure, these regions may, by
suffering a corresponding alteration, become too much
contracted to contain it; in which case it will extend into
the left hypochondric region, and may even occupy no
inconsiderable part of the umbilical region. This occurs
in females, whose chests are naturally contracted, or have
become so by the barbarous custom of tight lacing, and
from which more mischief has arisen, than from all the
dietetic errors which I shall have occasion to enumerate.

29. As the liver is connected with the diaphragm by
doublings of the peritonæum, termed *ligaments,* it follows
that, in the living subject, it will vary with respect to the
general cavity, in the acts of inspiration and expiration.

30. The figure of the liver is found to vary in different
animals, being generally determined by that of the animal
itself, or by that of the cavity in which it is contained.
In the human subject it is somewhat convex on its anterior
surface, irregular but concave on its posterior; it is extremely broad superiorly, but gradually becomes thinner
inferiorly, and terminates in a thin margin. Its surfaces
are smooth, being covered by the peritonæum, which forms
its several ligaments; viz. two, already mentioned, which
are attached to the diaphragm, and termed *lateral;* in the

middle of its lower and anterior margin is a *round* ligament adhering to the navel, through which the umbilical vein, &c. of the fœtus passes ; between this *round* ligament and the diaphragm is another, called the *suspensory ligament,* which adheres to the peritonæum of the anterior part of the abdomen. At the inferior edge of the liver there is a fissure extending some way up, particularly on its posterior surface, which divides it into two lobes of unequal size. These, from their situation in the abdominal cavity, are distinguished by the names of the right and left lobes, of which the right is the larger. Besides these, there is a smaller lobe, situated at the superior and posterior part, called, after its describer, *lobulus spigelii.* The liver usually weighs, in a middle-sized man, about three pounds twelve ounces.

31. In a depression on the concave surface of the right lobe, a pyriform-shaped bag, termed the *gall-bladder,* is lodged ; it has a duct terminating in the duodenum, through which the bile enters its cavity, and, at the same time, it constitutes the only outlet through which that fluid can return into the intestine.

32. The pyloric portion of the stomach is generally covered by the left lobe of the liver, and the gall-bladder would appear to rest usually on the duodenum.

33. The liver is composed of arteries, veins, nerves, lymphatics, and excretory ducts, united together by a peculiar parenchymatous structure. In every other gland in the body, the same blood which supplies it with nutrition is also adapted to its secretory office, and is conveyed to the organ by the same vessel ; but the liver requires *arterial* blood for its nourishment, and *venous* blood for the materials of its secretion ; the *hepatic* artery supplies the former, and the *vena portarum* conveys the latter. This vein is formed by the concurrence of all the veins of the abdominal viscera, which gather together and constitute one large trunk, called the *sinus* of the vena portarum,

which enters the liver, and divides in the manner of an artery. This peculiar arrangement induced some physiologists to suppose, that the bile was prepared in the abdominal viscera, or rather, that the blood underwent some peculiar modification in the intestines, which prepared it for the peculiar change it was destined to undergo in the liver; and they have supported this opinion by another equally gratuitous, that the blood of the vena portarum is better adapted for the secretion of bile, on account of the larger proportion of carbon and hydrogen which it must contain : but Bichat has observed, that fat, which is a highly hydrogenated fluid, does not require venous blood for its secretion ; and-contends, that the bile is secreted from the arterial blood of the liver, since the quantity of the latter sent to the liver is more in relation with the quantity of bile formed, than that of the venous blood ; and that the volume of the hepatic canal is not in proportion with that of the vena portarum. M. Majendie seems inclined to believe that both kinds of blood may serve in the secretion; he thinks that such a theory is indicated by anatomy ; for injections prove that all the vessels of the liver, arterial, venous, lymphatic, and excretory, communicate with each other. This idea, however, is highly repugnant to that simplicity which Nature observes in all her operations; and, although I am not prepared to prove that the blood of the vena portarum has more analogy with the bile than the arterial blood, still, the peculiar structure, disposition, and terminations of this singular vein appear to testify the important function it is destined to discharge. Dr. Saunders,* who has devoted much attention to the investigation of this subject, observes, that as the function of the vena portarum differs from that of other organs, so has it been

* A Treatise on the Structure, Economy, and Diseases of the Liver, by W. Saunders, M.D.

supposed to possess certain peculiarities of structure; but that the only marked difference consists in its tunic being thicker, in proportion to the capacity of its canal, than that of a common vein.

34. From the *sinus* of the vena portarum, three principal branches usually take their origin; these, by forming subordinate ramifications, in a regular series, at length arrive at their terminations, which are of two distinct kinds; the one with respect to the circulation of the blood; the other, as connected with their economy as secreting vessels. In the first point of view, they inosculate with branches of hepatic veins, and, through that channel, return to the inferior cava ⁺all that blood which is not employed in the business of secretion. It appears, therefore, that the hepatic veins are the common recipients of the contents of the hepatic artery, and likewise those of the vena portarum. The secreting termination of this vein is in the beginning of the hepatic ducts, which, Dr. Fordyce has observed, have improperly been called *pori biliarii;* for how can we, says he, with propriety call a tube of many inches in length a pore? These ducts must be exceedingly minute at their origin, since they preclude the admission of the red globules. They gradually enlarge by a union of branches, until at length they pass out from the liver, and form the trunk of the *hepatic duct.* From the side of this, rises another tube that leads into the gall-bladder, and the union of the two constitutes the common duct, or *ductus communis choledicus;* through which, it is obvious, that either the bile arising from the liver immediately, or that part of it which has stagnated for some time in the gall-bladder, may pass into the duodenum.

35. With respect to the chemical changes which the blood undergoes during its passage into bile, we are entirely ignorant; nor are we acquainted with any of the affinities by which the transmutation can be effected.

36. The liver is plentifully supplied with absorbents, which take their origin from every part of its substance, but more especially from the branches of the hepatic duct; this latter circumstance renders it probable that the bile looses a quantity of its aqueous particles as it passes through these passages, and changes from a dilute to a concentrated state.

37. The liver is supplied with nerves which arise principally from the *hepatic plexus*, and enter the substance of the liver with the hepatic artery.

38. M. Majendie states, that the secretion of bile appears constant; for, in whatever circumstances an animal is placed, if the orifice of the *ductus choledochus* is laid bare, this liquid is seen to flow, drop by drop, at the surface of the intestine; but we are not to conclude that, in the living body, its discharge into the duodenum is uniformly progressive, and without interruption: on the contrary, the termination of the duct will be occasionally pressed upon, during the peristaltic action of the intestine; at which periods, the duct will suffer a degree of distension, and the bile will find its way through the cystic duct into the gall-bladder. This effect will, in some measure, be promoted by the oblique manner in which the common duct perforates the intestine, although the more obvious utility of such an arrangement is to prevent the regurgitation of bile from the duodenum. To prevent the evils which must arise from a distended state of the gall-bladder, this viscus is so situated, as to be pressed upon by the stomach: I also entertain but little doubt that, in such a morbid condition of this receptacle, an irritation is communicated to the stomach, by which vomiting is produced, which must effectually contribute to the expulsion of its bile. M. Majendie has generally found it empty in animals that have died by the effect of an emetic poison. It seems very doubtful whether its coats are endowed with muscular powers to eject its contents.

39. Bile appears as a perfectly homogeneous fluid, of a yellowish green, or sometimes of a brown colour; in consistence, it is viscid and unctuous; its taste is bitter and pungent; and its odour peculiarly faint and nauseous. It is well known that the older chemists considered the bile as an animal soap, composed of soda and a resin; and this opinion received no small degree of support from the appearance of lather, which is produced by its agitation in a phial, and from that detergent quality so well known to every scourer of cloth. But in the present advanced state of science, the chemist is little disposed to infer the composition of a body from its external characters; he submits it to the ordeal of experiment, and tortures it, by the most refined operations; the happiest results have followed this rigorous process of inquiry. To the labours of Fourcroy, Thénard, and Berzelius, we are principally indebted for our knowledge of the composition of bile; and as the subject is one of deep interest to the physiologist and physician, I shall here give some account of their researches.

40. Boerhaave, by an extravagant error, regarded the bile as one of the most putrescible fluids; and hence originated many hypothetical and absurd theories on diseases and their treatment. Dr. Saunders has shewn, by a comparative experiment, that the bile of a healthy animal is far less disposed to putrify than its blood. The bile of the ox, from the greater quantity of it which may be procured, has been usually the subject of experiment. The odour, colour, and taste of bile appear to reside in a resinous matter, which is solid, very bitter, and, when pure, green; but when melted, it passes to yellow. It is soluble in alcohol and in pure alkalies; and is precipitable from the former by water, and from the latter by acids. The uncombined soda in bile does not exceed $\frac{1}{700}$ its weight; and, as this very minute quantity of alkali must be quite incapable of dissolving the large proportion of

resin which exists in bile, Thénard was induced to turn
his attention to the discovery of some other solvent of
resin, existing as a component part in that fluid. Acetate
of lead (the common sugar of lead of commerce) precipitates, he found, not only the resin, but the peculiar
substance, of which he was in search, in union with oxide
of lead. But an acetate, with a larger proportion of base,
(formed from eight parts of sugar of lead and one of
litharge,) produced a different effect, and precipitated only
the albumen and the resin. When the remaining liquid
was filtered, and the lead separated by means of sulphuretted hydrogen gas, it gave, on evaporation, a residue
having less bitterness and considerably more sweetness.
In this state the solvent of the resin could not be considered as pure, since it retained in solution a quantity
of acetate of soda, arising from the decomposition, by the
acetate of lead, of the salts of soda existing in the bile.
He again, therefore, precipitated the solution by the
acetate of lead saturated with oxide, and obtained an
insoluble compound of the peculiar matter and oxide of
lead. This was dissolved in vinegar; the oxide of lead
separated by sulphuretted hydrogen, and the acid driven
off by evaporation.

41. This substance, to which Thénard has given the
name of *picromel*, possesses the property of rendering the
resin of bile easily soluble in water. Three parts are
sufficient to one of the resin. The characters of *picromel*
are, that it is insoluble in water and alcohol, and incapable of being crystallised; that it precipitates nitrate of
mercury, and acetate of lead with excess of oxide; and
that it forms, with resin and a minute quantity of soda,
a triple compound, which is not decomposable by acids,
nor by alkaline or earthy salts. Chevallier has shewn
that it exists in human bile taken from the gall-bladder
after death, but he could not detect it in bile discharged

by vomiting.* It has been analysed by Dr. Thomson, who obtained products, indicating five atoms of carbon + three of oxygen + one of hydrogen.†

42. Besides picromel, there exists a peculiar principle in bile, to which the name of *yellow matter* has been given. It is precipitated by acids. It appears to be the source of those concretions which form in the gall-bladders of oxen, and which are valuable as a pigment, on account of the extreme beauty of their colour.

43. The composition of ox bile has been determined as follows : —

Water 700		
Resin.	24	
Picromel	60·5	
Yellow matter	4	*but variable.*
Soda	4	
Phosphate of soda.	2	
Muriate of soda.	3·2	
Sulphate of soda	0·8	
Phosphate of lime.	1·2	
Oxide of iron	*a trace.*	

$$\overline{800}$$

44. In analysing the bile of other animals, a similarity of composition was discovered, which little accords with the known diversity of their aliments; thus, that of the dog, the sheep, the cat, and the calf, was found to be precisely similar. The bile of the pig, on the contrary, contained neither *yellow matter* nor *picromel*. It consisted merely of resin in great quantity, of soda, and of salts, the nature of which has not been ascertained. It was entirely decomposed by acids, and even by the weakest — the acetic.

45. Berzelius is not disposed to regard the peculiar matter, which is considered to be *resin*, as strictly falling under that denomination : he says it is precipitable by

* Ann. de Chim. et Phys. ix. 400.   † Ann. of Phil. xiv. 70.

acids; and the precipitate is a compound of the acid employed with the green colouring matter of bile. This characteristic ingredient he calls *biliary* matter. He finds bile composed of

Water................907·4
Biliary matter............ 80·0
Mucus of the gall bladder .. 3·0
Alkalies and salts .... 9·6
_____
1000

One circumstance, adds M. Berzelius, relating to this biliary matter has much surprised me, which is, that it gives no ammonia by destructive distillation; therefore it contains no azote: but what can have become of the azote of the albuminous matter of the blood? for no vestige of it is found in any other of the constituent parts of the bile, nor does bile contain any ammonia.

46. M. Thénard also analysed human bile; and he is of opinion that his experiments have led him to as accurate a knowledge of it as of any other species. All the acids decompose it, and precipitate from it a large quantity of albumen and of resin. These may be separated from each other by alcohol. By the application of acetate of lead no *picromel* can be discovered; nor is any other ingredient found in human bile than yellow matter, albumen, resin, and salts. The proportions are the following :—

Water ....1000, or more.
Yellow matter, insoluble, and
   floating in the bile, a variable
   quantity from 2 to 10
Yellow matter in solution .... *a trace.*
Albumen 42
Resin 41
Soda........................ 5·6
Phosphates of soda and lime,
   sulphate and muriate of soda,
   and oxide of iron .... 4·5
_____
1100

47. The yellow matter appears to be, in every respect, similar to that of ox bile. The resin is yellowish; very fusible; bitter, but less so than that of ox bile; soluble in alcohol, from which it is precipitated by water; and soluble in alkalies, from which it is thrown down by acids. In water it appears scarcely to dissolve; and yet sulphuric and nitric acids occasion a precipitate from water which has been digested on it.

48. The *Pancreas,* vulgarly called the *sweet-bread,* is a large gland of the salivary kind, lying across the upper and back part of the abdomen, near the duodenum, behind the stomach, and between the liver and spleen. Its length is eight or nine inches, its breadth is about two fingers and a half, and its thickness about one finger : it generally weighs about three ounces. It is composed of innumerable small glands, the excretory ducts of which unite and form the pancreatic duct; which, in the human subject, always enters the duodenum with the ductus communis choledochus. Although the granulous structure of the pancreas has induced anatomists to regard it as a salivary gland, yet M. Majendie observes, that it differs in the smallness of the arteries which supply it, as well as in not appearing to receive any cerebral nerve. The peculiar fluid it secretes is, doubtless, necessary to digestion, but we are totally ignorant of the particular duty assigned to it. As we descend in the scale of animals, the pancreas disappears : it is found in the shark and skate, but in other fishes its place is supplied by *cecal appendices,* which afford a copious secretion analogous to the pancreatic liquor. The quantity of fluid prepared by this gland does not appear to bear a just proportion to its size. Dr. Fordyce first attempted to collect a quantity of it, by inserting a small quill into its duct, in a living dog; when there flowed out a colourless fluid, almost watery, having a saltish taste; and on letting it evaporate on a plate of glass, he observed crystals of common salt, and muriate of ammonia, together with a colourless mucilage. This ex-

periment, however, as its author candidly confesses, cannot
be considered as satisfactory, since the secretion did not
take place in its natural state; the quill might stimulate
the duct, and produce a different fluid. M. Majendie
employed a simpler mode; he laid bare the orifice of the
canal in a dog, wiped the surrounding mucous membrane
with a very fine cloth, and then waited until a drop of
liquid passed out; as soon as it appeared, he sucked it up
with a capillary tube; and in this manner he succeeded
in collecting some drops, but never enough to analyse it
with any precision : he recognised in it a slightly yellow
colour, a salt taste, but no odour; and he found that it
was alkaline, and partly coagulable by heat. The circumstance, says this able experimentalist, which most struck
me, was the smallness of its quantity ; a drop scarcely
passed out in half an hour, and I have sometimes waited
longer for it. That the pancreatic fluid plays an important
part in the elaboration of chyle, appears evident from the
fact, that diseases of that viscus are attended with extreme
emaciation.

49. The *Spleen* is a viscus of a deep blackish-red
colour, situated on the left hypochondrium, immediately
under the diaphragm, and above the kidney. Its figure
may be said to be that of a depressed oval, nearly twice as
long as it is broad, and almost twice as broad as it is
thick. However ingeniously we may speculate upon the
uses of this organ, nothing satisfactory has been hitherto
obtained upon the subject. It certainly does not appear
to be essential to life, for Mr. John Hunter removed it
from a wounded man, and the patient did well. Various
other instances of a similar kind stand on record. Hoffman
relates that, when the spleen is removed from dogs, they
rapidly increase in fatness. It cannot supply any fluid for
the digestive process, since it has no excretory duct. Some
have supposed, from the peculiarly dark livid colour of its
blood, and the difficulty with which it coagulates, that its

use is to produce some change upon the blood, in order
to adapt it for the secretion of bile. I think it very probable, from the relations which its blood-vessels bear to
those of the liver, that it administers, in some way or other,
to the latter viscus ; but it cannot be instrumental in the
formation of bile, as we have seen that this fluid can be
properly elaborated without. Is it not an organ of compensation, — a waste pipe, for the removal of any redundant
blood which may be thrown into the liver ? or a reservoir,
to supply any deficiency which circumstances may create ?
and that, in this respect, it is to its sanguiferous, what the
gall-bladder is to its biliary system ?

50. Having completed the history of the glands destined for the secretion of the several fluids which are
essential to the digestive process, I shall pause a short
time, in order to offer a few observations upon the nature
of those wonderful phenomena, which arise, as it were, on
the doubtful confines of chemistry and vitality. What is
secretion ? How are we to explain the fact of blood being
successively converted into saliva, gastric juice, bile, and a
variety of other equally dissimilar fluids, by its mere transmission through a series of minute tubes ? If we direct
our attention to the most simple form of secretion, termed
serous exhalation, we shall hastily arrive at the conclusion,
that a separation of the thinner from the thicker parts of
the blood is all that has been effected by the operation,
and that the organs by which the several membranes are
thus supplied, are consequently mere *sieves ;* for if we examine the composition of the fluid secreted by the serous
membranes, it will appear to be the serum of the blood,
deprived of a certain quantity of albumen. The following
very interesting observations by M. Majendie prove that
the physical disposition of the small vessels has an influence upon the exhalation. When, in the dead body,
tepid water is injected into an artery that goes into a

serous membrane, as soon as the current is established
from the artery to the vein, a great number of small drops
pass out of the membrane, and quickly evaporate. This
phenomenon has certainly a close analogy with exhalation.
If we employ a solution of gelatine, coloured with vermilion, to inject a whole body, it frequently happens that
the gelatine is deposited round the circumvolutions, and
in the cerebral anfractuosities, without the colouring matter having escaped from the vessels; on the contrary, the
whole injection spreads at the external and internal surface
of the *choroid*. If linseed oil be used, coloured also by
vermilion, the oil, deprived of the colouring matter, is
often seen deposited in the great synovial capsule of arti-
culations; whilst there is no transudation at the surface of
the brain, nor in the interior of the eye. With such results
before me, and observing, at the same time, that the structure of all glands agrees in this fact, that they are composed
of vessels of infinitely small diameter, I am bound to conclude, that one part, at least, of the process of secretion is
mechanical, and that whatever other office a gland may
perform, that it undoubtedly acts as a sieve or filter. The
discoveries which modern chemists have effected, with
regard to the atomic composition of bodies, seem to me to
be capable of being brought, in some degree, to bear on
the question before us. It appears probable that the ultimate, as well as proximate atoms of different bodies, are
endowed with different degrees of magnitude: a cracked
jar has been known to retain oxygen for a considerable
period, without contamination; but when the same jar
was filled with hydrogen, this latter gas speedily escaped:
we find a rational explanation of this fact in the supposition, that the atoms of hydrogen have less magnitude than
those of oxygen. Again, if diluted alcohol be kept in a
vessel carefully closed by a slip of bladder, after some time
the spirit will be found stronger; whence it appears, that
the alcoholic vapour transpires through this animal mem-

brane less freely than aqueous vapour: are then the atoms
of water smaller than those of alcohol? Let us consider
this question: an atom of water is compounded of one
atom of oxygen and one atom of hydrogen; whereas an
atom of alcohol consists of two atoms of carbon, one atom
of oxygen, and three atoms of hydrogen: but it may be
said, that bodies chemically combined cannot be thus disunited by mechanical division: this, as a general proposition, is undoubtedly true; but we have ample proofs to
shew that chemical affinities may be suspended in the
living body. In reflecting upon all the circumstances and
bearings of this important and interesting subject, I have
often been struck with the wisdom and extreme simplicity
of the process by which the blood is separated by the
structure of the eye, into those parts which are of such
striking utility in its economy. It was essential that the
crystalline humour should be perfectly transparent, and
that the interior surface of the choroid coat should be
impregnated with a dark pigment, in order to absorb the
light immediately after it has traversed the retina; now,
if we submit the matter of the lens to analysis, we shall
find that it coagulates by boiling, and has all the chemical
properties of the colouring matter of blood, except colour,
which is entirely absent. What then has become of this
colouring ingredient? we shall find that it has been appropriated by the vessels of the choroid, for the important
purpose above stated. On examining this pigment, its
composition will be found to confirm such a theory; for,
when dried and ignited, it will burn as easily as a vegetable
substance, and the ash will contain much iron. For these
results we are indebted to the labours of Berzelius; and
they certainly shew that the circulating blood is decomposed on the interior surface of the choroid, leaving there
its colouring matter, and conveying the remainder to the
inner part of the eye perfectly limpid and colourless.

51. But filtration cannot explain the development of

those secreted fluids which contain proximate principles that do not exist in the blood ; — no foreign ingredient is added, no chemical reagent is interposed, and yet the fluid which flows from the organised laboratory has acquired chemical properties, which render it decidedly different from the common circulating mass. The agent in this case can only be the nervous fluid, which appears to exert its influence principally upon the albumen, which M. Berzelius considers as the source * of every substance that peculiarly characterises each secretion : all the other parts are contained in the blood, and are identical with the fluid separated from the serum after its coagulation.

52. Every attempt to understand the manner in which the nervous fluid produces the phenomena of secretion, has hitherto completely failed; the changes to which it gives origin no art can imitate, nor any philosophy explain; but, although we are thus unable to trace the steps of nature, we may venture to inquire into the general direction of the path which she follows. It must be allowed that a considerable analogy subsists between the operations of the nervous fluid, as an agent of secretion, and that of galvanic electricity; they both suspend the natural affinities of bodies, dissever elements between which the strongest attractions exist, and determine them to unite in different forms and proportions. In illustration of this truth, the following ingenious experiment of Dr. Wollaston may be introduced : — he took a glass tube, two inches long, and three-quarters of an inch in diameter, and closed one of its extremities with a piece of bladder; he then poured a little water into the tube, with $\frac{1}{240}$ parts of its weight of common salt; he wetted the bladder on

---

* Our English chemist, Mr. Hatchett, expressed the same opinion, in a paper published in the Philosophical Transactions for 1800 : he there shews that it is convertible into *gelatine* and *fibrine*. Is not the chick produced in the egg from the albumen?

the outside, and placed it on a piece of silver; he then
bent a zinc wire, so that one of its ends touched the silver,
and the other entered the tube the length of an inch:
in the same instant, the external face of the bladder gave
indications of the presence of pure soda; so that, under
the influence of this very weak electricity, there was a
decomposition of muriate of soda, and a passage of the
soda, separated from the acid, through the bladder. It
seems rational to believe that something analogous may
happen in the act of secretion. Dr. Young has developed
this idea still farther; and has observed, that we may
easily imagine that, at the subdivision of a minute artery,
a nervous filament may pierce it on one side, and afford
a pole positively electrical, and another opposite filament a
negative one; then the particles of oxygen and nitrogen
contained in the blood being most attracted by the positive pole, will tend towards the branch which is nearest to
it, while those of the hydrogen and carbon will take the
opposite channel; and that both these portions may be
again subdivided, if it be required; and the fluid thus
analysed may be recombined into new forms by a reunion
of a certain number of each of the kinds of minute ramifications.

III. VESSELS FOR CARRYING THE NUTRITIVE PRO-
DUCT TO THE CURRENT OF THE CIRCULATION.

53. The *Lacteals*, so called from the milky appearance
of the liquor they are destined to carry, arise, by number-
less open mouths, from the inner surface of the intestines.
Each lacteal takes its origin upon one of the villi, by
numerous short radiated branches, and each branch is
furnished with an orifice for imbibing the chyle. The
radiated branches are collected into fasciculi, which are
enclosed in processes of the inner coat of the intestines.

These fasciculi are of a roundish form, and have been called *ampullulæ* of Leiberkuhn, from the author considering them as little bottles receiving the chyle. From the villi, the lacteals run a considerable way under the muscular coat of the intestines, and then pass obliquely through it, uniting in their course into larger branches. Upon the surface of the intestines an external set appears; it runs between the peritoneal and muscular coats, and commonly proceeds some way in the direction of the intestine, and with few ramifications. The superficial and deep-seated lacteals communicate freely in the substance of the intestines: those of the *jejunum* are larger and more numerous than those of the *ilium*, the principal part of the chyle being contained in the former. The absorbents of the *great*, are proportionally of an inferior size to those of the *small* intestines, and have seldom, though sometimes, been observed to be filled with chyle. In their course they pass through a great number of lacteal or *mesenteric* glands, which, like the lacteals themselves, are largest and most numerous in that part of the mesentery which belongs to the jejunum.

54. The *Mesenteric Glands* are seated in the fat, between the layers of the mesentery, near the branches of the blood-vessels. They are commonly scattered over the mesentery, at a little distance from each other; but there are seldom any observed within two or three inches of the intestines. They differ from each other in size, some being about half or two-thirds of an inch in diameter, while others are so small as to be traced with difficulty. Their structure is the same as that of the absorbent glands in other parts of the body, but they are generally flatter, and are of a pale colour. When filled with chyle, they are nearly as white as the fluid contained in them. The lacteals having passed through these glands, proceed forward, and by anastomosing form a set of trunks, which, together with those of the lymphatics, unite and constitute

the *thoracic duct,* which ultimately opens into the sub-clavian vein. Much discussion has arisen as to the mechanism by which the chyle is made to pass forward through the lacteal system : capillary attraction would appear to have some influence in the operation, since ab-sorption continues after death ; during life, the pressure of the abdominal muscles, and the pulsation of the arteries, no doubt contribute to the effect. In the interior of the thoracic duct, and in the lacteals, there exist valves so disposed as to permit the fluid to pass forward towards the subclavian vein, but to prevent its return.

IV. The Lungs.

55. Although the lungs perform several essential ope-rations not immediately connected with nutrition, still, as the chyle is incapable of becoming blood without their assistance, they necessarily constitute an important link in the chain of digestive functions. It would be digressing too much from the plan of this work, to enter into ana-tomical details of their structure ; but it may be necessary to remind the practitioner, that the lungs are supplied with a part of the nerve of the eighth pair, and some fila-ments of the sympathetic, which will account for the sym-pathies which subsist between the respiratory and digestive organs.*

V. The Kidneys.

56. These organs are situated upon the sides of the vertebral column, just before the last false ribs. From

---

* Upon this subject, the practitioner will do well to consult the highly ingenious paper by Mr. Charles Bell, published in the Philosophical Transactions, and entitled, " *On the Nerves; giving an Account of some Experiments on their Structure and Functions, which lead to a new Arrangement of the System.*"

their oblong figure, they have been compared in shape to large beans. The right kidney lies under the great lobe of the liver, and is consequently lower than the left, which lies under the spleen. Their volume is small when compared with the large quantity of fluid which they secrete; and it appears probable, that the chemical functions which they perform are less extensive than those which may be regarded as more strictly mechanical. They are generally surrounded with a considerable quantity of fat: their parenchyma is composed of two substances; the one exterior, vascular, or *cortical;* the other, called *tubular,* disposed in a certain number of cones, the bases of which correspond to the surface of the organ, while their summits unite in the membranous cavity called *pelvis.* These cones appear to be formed by a great number of small hollow fibres, which are excretory canals of a particular kind, and which are generally filled with urine. It is a curious fact, that if a slight compression be made upon these uriniferous cones, the urine will pass out in considerable quantity; but, instead of being limpid, as when it passes out naturally, it is muddy and thick, which evidently proves that the hollow fibres act as filters. In respect to its volume, no organ receives so much blood as the kidney: the artery which is directed there is large, short, and proceeds immediately from the aorta. Haller has decided, that no less than a thousand ounces of blood may pass through the renal structure in the space of an hour: and the extreme facility with which the coarsest injections pass through the renal arteries into the *ureters,* or excretory ducts, affords a convincing proof of the immediate connexion which exists between all the different parts of the structure of the kidney. The filaments of the great sympathetic are alone distributed to these organs.

VI. The Skin.

57. The skin forms the envelope of the body, and is lost in the mucous membranes at the entrance of all the cavities; although some assert that these membranes are only a continuation of it, and thus account for the sympathy which subsists between such structures. Be this as it may, it is evident that the interior organs, especially the stomach, alimentary canal, the lungs, the liver, and the kidneys, sympathise in a very remarkable degree with the surface of the body. So striking and constant is the sympathy between these latter organs and the skin, that they appear capable of reciprocally assisting each other in their operations : where cold contracts the pores of the surface, we find the kidneys excited to a greater degree of activity ; and changes in the secretions of the skin are attended with corresponding alterations in the urinary discharge. Its sympathy with the stomach is also evinced by the phenomena which accompany digestion. It has been ascertained by Lavoisier and Seguin, that the cutaneous transpiration is at its minimum during chymification, and at its maximum after its completion.

58. According to M. Thénard, the liquid that escapes from the skin is composed of a great deal of water, a small quantity of acetic acid, of muriates of soda and potass, a small proportion of earthy phosphate, an atom of oxide of iron, and a trace of animal matter: the skin exhales also carbonic acid.

59. Much controversy has existed with regard to the absorbing powers of the skin; but the question appears to me to have been settled by the experiments of M. Seguin ; and that, as long as the epidermis remains entire, substances in contact with the surface will not pass into the circulation, but that as soon as it is abraded, absorption takes place. If, however, friction is employed, an effect follows

which simple application would not produce ; it cannot be doubted that mercury and other bodies may be thus made to pass into the system. This question is one of great importance, inasmuch as it enables us to appreciate the value of nourishing baths of milk, broth, &c.

60. I have thus, with as much brevity as the subject would allow, offered a sketch of the different organs by which aliment is converted into blood. My object has been to bring into one point of view all those facts which are capable of practical application, and to exclude, as far as possible, those which have no other than theoretical relations to the subject before us. Minute anatomy is of little service to the physician, but without a knowledge of the positions and localities of the different organs which constitute the seats of the diseases he may be called upon to cure, he will be inevitably led into error. In consequence of such deficiency, a practitioner at once refers a fulness of the right epigastrium to the liver, forgetting that a distended state of the duodenum may account for the symptom; in like manner, he will attribute to the kidney, pains which ought to be referred to the posterior edge of the liver. A hundred parallel examples might be adduced, but those I have stated will answer the purpose of illustration.

PHYSIOLOGICAL HISTORY OF DIGESTION.

NUTRITION :—*its final Cause.*— *Old Age:* — *Sir A. Carlisle's View of the Disorders of Senility objectionable.—
The Author's Opinion. — Chemical and Mechanical
Agents of Digestion.— Conventional acceptation of the
term Chemical.— Mastication.— Insalivation.— Erro-
neous Opinion of Dr. Fordyce and others with respect
to the Use of the Saliva.—Deglutition. — Action of the
Gastric Juice.—* CHYMIFICATION :—*Artificial Diges-
tion.— Office of the Pylorus.— Vomiting.— Duodenal
Digestion.—* CHYLIFICATION : — *Uses of the Bile. —
Mr. Brodie's Experiments. — Chemical Nature of the
Chyle: — its Absorption.— Excrementitious Matter.—*
LIQUID ALIMENTS :—*how decomposed in the Stomach.
— The liquid part absorbed or coagulated. — Digestion
of Milk, Broth, Wine, Oil, &c.— Lymphatic Absorption.—* SANGUIFICATION.—RESPIRATION. —*Practical Conclusions. — Urinary Secretion. — Acidifying
Powers of the Kidney.—The Quality of Urine influenced
by the Digestive Process.—Necessity of Urinary Secretion.—A general View of the Digestive Process.—Reasons for believing in the existence of an Agent analogous
to Electricity.— Experiments of Dr. Wilson Philip.—
Speculations of the Author.*

61. A very superficial examination of an organised body
will convince us, that it is constantly losing portions of the
matter of which it is composed : several of its organs are
incessantly engaged in separating fluids, which are loaded
with its more solid constituents : and it is on the necessity
of repairing these habitual losses, that the want of aliment
is founded ; while the identification of such nutritive
materials with the composition of the organs which they

are destined to supply, constitutes N U T R I T I O N. And with
such nicety are these processes of waste and repair ad-
justed, that, whatever may be the quantity of food taken,
or however the circumstances under which it is consumed
may vary, the same individual, after having augmented in
weight in proportion to the quantity of ingesta, will return,
in the space of twenty-four hours, to nearly the same
standard, provided he is not growing, nor has suffered any
disorder of function. During this period the food has been
decomposed, and re-combined into compounds analogous
to those which compose the organs to which it is carried :
and this appears to take place with the same facility, however remote the composition of the aliment may be from
that of the substances with which it assimilated. Living
bodies, then, have not inaptly been compared to furnaces,
into which inert substances are successively thrown, which
combine amongst themselves in various manners, maintain
a certain place, and perform an action determined by the
nature of the combinations they have formed, and at last
fly off, in order to become again subject to the laws of
inanimate nature. These views naturally suggest several
important questions for our consideration. If every part
of the machine be thus capable of immediate and constant
repair, why should it ever wear out ? Does there exist
some secret spring which is incapable of renewal, and at
whose expense all the subordinate parts of the machinery
are kept in repair? And why should life be terminated
by the hardening of fibres, and the obstruction of vessels,
when those very fibres and vessels are susceptible of
renewal? These are mysteries which cannot be cleared
up until the sealed fountain of vitality be laid open. It
seems probable, that every individual has a certain measure
of living energy assigned to him, and which is gradually
expended in directing and maintaining the performance of
certain functions : when this is exhausted, the individual
must perish, for it is incapable of renewal. Sir A. Carlisle,

in his work on the Disorders of Old Age, remarks, that it
seems little better than a vulgar error, to consider the termination of advanced life as the inevitable consequence of
time, when the immediate cause of death in old persons
is generally known to be some well-marked disease. I
have directed some attention to this subject, and I feel
warranted by experience to state, that the greater number
of those who terminate their existence at an advanced age,
die from the exhaustion of vital power in some one of their
principal organs, the consequence of which is an ill-marked
species of inflammation. Symptoms indicating the existence of peritonitis are by no means uncommon ; in some
cases, the lungs or the brain appear to be the seats of
disease. The arterial system owes its regularity of action
to the presiding influence of the nervous power ; and if this
be withdrawn, or irregularly supplied, inflammation follows.
It is to such a cause that the local congestions, and topical
inflammations, which so frequently occur in fever, are to
be entirely attributed. With all due respect, therefore, for
the experience and skill of the author to whom I allude, I
must differ with him in the view he has taken of the disorders of senility : the doctrine he inculcates is dangerous,
and may lead to practical mischief. In cases of congestion,
blood-letting is undoubtedly a judicious remedy, when
directed with measured caution, because it removes an
effect which may contribute to aggravate the original
disease, or to obstruct the sanative operations which
nature institutes for her own relief ; but we should perfectly understand the mode in which it operates, and not
mistake secondary for primary diseases.

62. Although these views may disparage every effort
to prolong the natural term of existence, they afford us
the satisfaction of knowing that we may ward off those
accidents which would otherwise lead to its premature
termination. Although we cannot augment the allotted
measure of our vital energy, we can, at least, learn to hus-

band its resources, and not to consume, with wanton indifference, the unrecruitable oil by which the lamp of life
is supported.

63. In examining the phenomena of waste and supply,
we shall observe that there is a marked difference, depending on age, health, temperament, and bodily exercise, in
the proportion of the parts which enter into this current,
and of those which abandon it; and that the velocity of
the motions usually varies according to the different conditions of each living being. A knowledge of these differences, which is to be discovered only by ample experience and well-directed observation, must constitute the
basis of a true theory for the regulation of diet. If it be
said, that a deficient quantity of food is indicated by our
feelings, and that an excess is carried off without inconvenience, I shall reply, that nature rarely suffers from
abstinence, but continually from repletion ; that while in
one case she limits her expenditure to meet the exigencies
of her income, in the other, she is called upon to exercise
an injurious liberality to throw off the useless burden. In
the vigour of health and youth, this expenditure is not
felt; but the period will assuredly arrive when it must be
repaid with compound interest.

64. If *chemical* change be defined that change of composition in which the elements of bodies are differently
arranged, with regard to their proportions and modes of
combination, the conversion of aliment into blood strictly
falls under that description ; but the definition generally
includes the operation of certain known laws, by which
such changes are produced. In this latter sense the
analogy fails us ; for the forces which determine the decomposition of food, and its recombination into chyle, are
undoubtedly not to be measured or appreciated by the laws
which govern the transmutations of inanimate matter :
we may, nevertheless, conventionally retain the term, in
order to distinguish such actions from those which are

more strictly mechanical; and, although, in the progress
of such discussions, we may lapse into the common language of chemistry, the reader will, from this explanation,
readily understand the latitude with which it is to be
received.

65. In every change which the aliment undergoes, from
its introduction into the mouth to the exclusion of its
refuse, and the perfect assimilation of its nutritive part
with the blood, we shall discover the combined operation
of chemical and mechanical agents. When the food enters
the mouth, it is at once submitted to the mechanical process of division by the teeth; and, during its mastication,
it becomes intimately mixed and combined with a chemical solvent, which prepares it for the process which it
has shortly to undergo in the stomach. The quantity of the
salivary secretion appears to be augmented by the pressure
occasioned upon the glands by the act of mastication; but
its flow, although perhaps less in quantity, equally takes
place without the aid of such pressure, as is proved by
the phenomena observed during the repast of the criminal
already alluded to (24). The glands appointed to secrete this
fluid seem to act in sympathy with those of the stomach,
both of which are simultaneously excited by the stimulus
of the food, or even by the contemplation of a favourite
meal.   Macbride considered the saliva as a ferment.   The
ground of this opinion arose from his having made experiments, in which pieces of meat and water were mixed
together, alone in one vessel, and in another the same
substances were mixed with saliva : in the former case no
bubbles of air were perceptible, but in the latter a copious
evolution of them took place.   This, however, was a fallacy, depending upon the viscidity, which the saliva imparted to the water, retaining the escape of air until it
became sensible.   Dr. Fordyce, on the other hand, con-
tends, that the saliva answers no other purpose than to
lubricate the passages through which the food is to pass,

because he cannot discover in the composition of that fluid any ingredients which are likely to act as powerful solvents. But the processes of nature are more refined than those of art; and where chemistry refuses its aid, we may often derive information from simple experience. This happens in the question before us: the introduction of saliva into the stomach is obviously essential to a healthy digestion. That a dry state of the fauces should be attended with loss of appetite, may, perhaps, be reconciled on the supposition that the salivary glands sympathise with those of the stomach, and that therefore such a condition of the fauces is merely indicative of a deranged state of the gastric secretion; but this explanation will not apply to those cases of anorexia, in which the saliva is duly secreted, but is, from some mechanical cause, not swallowed. Ruysch knew a man who was wholly deprived of his appetite by a fistula in one of the salivary ducts; and it is well known to the physician who has attended maniacal patients, that the constant spitting in which such persons occasionally indulge, is invariably attended with loss of appetite, dyspepsia, and emaciation. Insalivation, therefore, is as essential as mastication; and although it will not supersede the necessity of this latter operation, as we find that persons who do not chew their food have often, on that account, a laborious digestion, yet it may, to a certain degree, compensate for it; and it is probable that the abundance of saliva in children may render mastication less necessary. The change which the savour and odour of food undergo in the mouth, sufficiently testifies some chemical action; but it must, at the same time, be admitted, that the deglutition is assisted by the moisture and lubrication which the saliva affords.

66. M. Majendie says, we are informed that mastication and insalivation are carried sufficiently far by the degree of resistance and savour of the food; besides, the sides of the mouth being endowed with *tact*, and the

tongue with a real sense of *touch*, they are very capable
of appreciating the physical changes which the food
undergoes. Though deglutition is very simple in appearance, it is nevertheless the most complicated of all the
muscular actions that serve for digestion. It is produced
by the contraction of a great number of muscles, and
requires the concurrence of many important organs. It
has been divided into three periods : in the first, the food
passes from the mouth to the pharynx ; in the second, it
passes the opening of the glottis, that of the nasal canals,
and arrives at the œsophagus ; in the third, it passes
through this tube, and enters the stomach. The progress
of the alimentary bolus is facilitated by mucus, which is
pressed out of the follicles over which it passes. Its passage through the œsophagus appears to be comparatively
slow, and it sometimes stops for several seconds : every
person must be convinced of this fact from his own sensations ; and where the bolus has been very large, its passage
has been accompanied with vivid pain, occasioned by the
distension of the nervous filaments which surround the
pectoral portion of the canal.

67. When the aliment is introduced into the stomach,
it appears to remain there a short period before it undergoes any change ; but this varies according to its nature,
and other circumstances. It has been stated (12), that
although the stomach is a single bag, it may be considered,
with respect to its functions, as divisible into two distinct
cavities, the one termed the *pyloric,* the other the *splenic*
extremity ; * and these portions are, during the activity of
the stomach, separated from each other by a peculiar
muscular contraction. They evidently appear to perform
different offices in the process of digestion. The splenic

* In the horse, the mucous membrane of the two extremities of the
stomach has a striking difference of structure : the horse being a graminivorous animal, this arrangement may, in some degree, perhaps, answer
the purpose of the more complicated stomachs of the *ruminantia.*

portion would seem to separate from the food the superfluous quantity of water, and then to transmit it to the
pyloric division, where it undergoes the first great alimentary change, or is converted into *chyme*: during this
operation, both orifices of the stomach are closed. I shall
not consume the time of the reader by relating the
numerous theories of putrefaction, concoction, fermentation, and trituration, which have been suggested by physiologists of different ages, to account for the changes
which the food undergoes : it will be sufficient to state,
that this question is at length determined, and that the
solvent energy of the peculiar liquid, which has been
already described (25) under the appellation of *gastric
juice*, together with the motions of the stomach, alone
produce that change upon the aliment which we have
next to consider.

68. It is not easy to define the exact nature of *chyme*:
but authors agree in considering it a homogeneous paste,
greyish, of a sweetish taste, slightly acid, and retaining
some of the properties of the food. M. Majendie has lately
examined the subject with greater precision, and it follows
from his experiments, that there are as many species of
chyme as there are varieties of food; if, at least, we may
judge by colour, consistence, and sensible qualities.

69. The *gastric juice* is remarkable for three qualities,—
a coagulating (25), antiputrescent, and solvent power. I
have already spoken of its coagulating properties. Of its
antiseptic powers abundant proofs have been furnished by
the experiments of several physiologists. Dr. Fordyce
found that the most putrid meat, after remaining a short
time in the stomach of a dog, became perfectly sweet.
Spallanzani ascertained that the gastric juice of the crow
and the dog will preserve veal and mutton, and without
loss of weight, for thirty-seven days in winter; whereas,
the same meats, immersed in water, emit a fetid smell as
early as the seventh day, and by the thirtieth, are resolved

into a state of most offensive putridity. The solvent powers of the stomach are equally remarkable. Reaumur and Spallanzani enclosed pieces of the toughest meats, and of the hardest bones, in small perforated tin cases, to guard against the effects of muscular action, and then introduced them into the stomach of a buzzard : the meats were uniformly found diminished to three-fourths of their bulk in the space of twenty-four hours, and reduced to slender threads, and the bones were wholly digested, either upon the first trial, or a few repetitions of it. To ascertain whether the chymification of food were entirely attributable to this gastric solvent, experiments were instituted in order to produce what has been termed *artificial digestion.* After having macerated food, Spallanzani mixed it with gastric juice, and then exposed it, in a tube, to a temperature equal to that of the stomach : it is said that the experiment succeeded, and that *chyme* was produced. M. de Montegre, however, has shewn the fallacy of this conclusion; but, says M. Majendie, we are not to conclude, from the failure of such an experiment, that the same fluid cannot dissolve the food when it is introduced into the stomach. The circumstances are indeed far from being the same ; in the stomach, the temperature is constant, the food is pressed and agitated, and the saliva and gastric juice are constantly renewed; as soon as the chyme is formed it is carried away, — circumstances which do not occur in a tube containing a mixture of the food and gastric juice. It seems probable that the gastric juice remains on the surface of the stomach, and is secreted as the digestion proceeds. The chymification of the food commences on its surface, and gradually proceeds towards its centre: a soft layer may be easily detached, which presents the appearance of a corroded and half-dissolved substance. The white of a hard egg, for instance, very shortly assumes an appearance like that which would be produced upon it by immersion in vinegar, or an alkaline solution. This change, if duly

performed, is not accompanied with any notable extrication
of gas ; but, should the vital powers of the stomach be
deficient, a different species of decomposition takes place,
the laws of chemistry gain the ascendancy, and results are
produced more or less analogous to those which would
arise from the same materials, if placed under similar circumstances of temperature and motion, in a vessel out of
the body.

70. Whatever may be the alimentary substance introduced, the chyme will present the invariable property of
reddening paper coloured with turnsol, and it has always
a sharp odour and taste.

71. The period necessary for chymification must vary
according to the nature and volume of the food, the degree
of mastication and insalivation it may have previously
undergone, and the degree of vital energy possessed by
the stomach. The whole of the aliment is not simultaneously converted, but portions, as they are perfected, are
successively passed out of the stomach into the duodenum,
there to undergo farther changes, to be presently described.
In this case, the *pylorus* must, as its name implies, be
endowed with a peculiar sensibility and vigilance, by
which it is enabled to distinguish between the crude and
chymified portions, so as to admit the latter, while it
opposes the passage of the former. To this theory it has
been objected, that various foreign bodies have been known
to pass from the stomach into the intestines, as buttons,
pieces of iron, &c.; but it must be remembered, that such
substances may be even less irritating than crude food,
and that they are, besides, not admitted into the intestines
until they have been frequently presented to the pylorus, and
the sensibility of this valve has been diminished. Nature
has endowed the eye with an irritability which instantly
causes it to close upon the contact of an extraneous substance ; but the oculist who is in the habit of performing
operations on that organ, knows that, after the instrument

has touched the eye several times, its irritability ceases, and it becomes passive. M. Majendie, however, expresses his scepticism with regard to this elective power of the pylorus. He seems to consider the idea as fanciful; but I would ask whether there is any thing improbable in the supposition? Is not every part of the machine endowed with a sensibility adapted to the office it is destined to perform? The eye is stimulated by light, the heart by blood; and why may we not suppose that the pylorus is, in a like manner, stimulated by the contact of chyme? If we reject this idea, can we propose a less objectionable explanation of the phenomena?—certainly not: on the contrary, the whole economy of the stomach is adverse to any other belief. If an unnatural stimulus be given to this viscus, so as to increase its motions, with a view of accelerating the progress of its contents into the duodenum, before they have been duly converted, what happens? The pylorus refuses its assent to their egress, and the motions of the stomach are inverted, so as to expel the crude food by vomiting.

72. In order to facilitate the expulsion of chyme through the pylorus, numerous glands are placed around it, which furnish a lubricating fluid. For the same purpose, glands are found in the crops of birds, near the entrance into the gizzard. In the human subject, we recognise a similar provision in the lower part of the rectum, in order to assist the alvine evacuation.

73. After the chyme has passed into the duodenum, it becomes mixed and incorporated with the peculiar fluid secreted by that intestine; it still, however, preserves its colour, its semi-fluid consistence, its sharp odour, and its slightly acid savour, until it reaches the sacculated angle, where it meets with the biliary and pancreatic fluids, with which it mixes, and undergoes an important chemical change, which has been very accurately examined by M. Majendie; and as the results of his inquiry are capable of throwing

some light upon the subject, I shall offer a summary view
of them. As soon as the chyme mingles with the chylopoietic fluids, it assumes a yellow colour and a bitter taste,
and its sharp odour is diminished ; but those changes, as
well as the phenomena which accompany them, are variable, and appear to be influenced by the quality of the
food. If the chyme proceed from animal or vegetable
matters containing fat or oil, irregular filaments, sometimes
flat, and at other times rounded, are seen to form here and
there on its surface, and to attach themselves quickly to
the *valvulæ conniventes.* They appear to consist of crude
chyle. This matter, however, was not observed when the
aliment did not contain fat : in the latter case, the product
appears as a greyish layer, more or less thick, adhering to
the mucous membrane, and may possibly contain only the
elements of chyle. This change, whatever may be its
chemical nature, is evidently produced by the action of
the biliary and pancreatic liquids, aided by the agitation,
or *churning,* which the substances undergo by the motions
of the duodenum itself, as well as by that communicated
to it from the colon, to which it is attached.

74. Various opinions have existed, with regard to the
use of the bile : some physiologists have considered it as
merely excrementitious, and with this opinion the general
mass of mankind would appear to coincide; for there is
scarcely a patient who does not complain of being tormented with bile, while the shop of the druggist groans
with the weight of pills which are calculated to expel this
fearful enemy from the system. The situation alone of
the liver, connected as it is, in every instance, with the
upper part of the alimentary canal, would be sufficient
to repel such an idea. Others have imagined, that it
is a natural and habitual stimulus to the intestines, keeping up their energy and peristaltic motions. It cannot be
denied that this is one of its secondary uses ; it likewise,
from its saponaceous and soluble qualities, diminishes the

adhesive nature of the fæces, and, by smoothing their surfaces, promotes their evacuation ; but its first and most
important use is to change the nutritive part of the *chyme*
into a new and more highly animalised product, termed
chyle, and to separate from it the useless and excrementitious part.   That such is the truth, is at once proved by
the fact, that *chylification* takes place just at the part
where the bile flows into the intestine ; nothing like chyle
is ever found in the stomach ; and Dr. Prout, whose able
researches in animal chemistry are well known, has ascertained that albumen, which is the characteristic part of
chyle, is never to be discovered in herbivorous animals
higher than the pylorus.   The question is, moreover, set
at rest by the experimental inquiries of Mr. Brodie.   He
tied a ligature round the common duct of a cat, so as completely to prevent the entrance of the bile into the intestine ; he then noted the effects produced in the digestion
of the food which the animal had swallowed, either immediately before, or after the operation.   The experiment
was repeated several times, and the results were uniform.
The production of chyme took place as usual, but the
conversion of chyme into chyle was invariably and completely interrupted.   Not the smallest trace of this latter
fluid was discoverable, either in the intestines or in the
lacteals.   The former contained a semi-fluid substance,
resembling the chyme found in the stomach, with this difference, that it became of a thicker consistence, in proportion as it was at a greater distance from the stomach, and
that, as it approached the termination of the ilium, the fluid
part of it had altogether disappeared, and there remained
only a solid substance, differing in appearance from ordinary fæces.   The lacteals contained a transparent fluid,
which probably consisted partly of lymph, partly of the
more fluid parts of the chyme which had been absorbed.
These experiments, then, clearly demonstrate, that the
office of the bile is to change the nutritive part of the

chyme into chyle, and to separate from it the excrementitious matter. How, then, it may be asked, does it happen, that persons live for a considerable period, in whom the flow of bile into the duodenum is interrupted? The truth is, that the obstruction of the duct by disease is seldom so complete as to prevent the passage of bile altogether, and the white appearance of the fæces may prove the deficiency, or morbid condition, but not the total absence of bile. To ascertain how far this supposition might be supported by experiment, I poured some dilute muriatic acid upon a portion of fæces that was perfectly white, when a green colour was immediately produced, which could not have happened without the presence of bile.

75. In the few authenticated cases of the total obliteration of the duct, the emaciation has been extreme, and the circumstance of the patient having lived a few weeks or months, under such circumstances, only proves that nutrition may take place, to some extent, without any chyle being formed. In the above experiments of Mr. Brodie, it appeared that the more fluid parts of the chyme had been absorbed; and probably this would have been sufficient to maintain life for a limited period, especially where but little exhaustion had been occasioned by exercise. We know that nutritive glysters will afford support, and yet we are quite certain that no chyle can be formed under such circumstances. Sir E. Home has related the case of a child in which no gall ducts existed. The child did not live long, but appears to have died rather of a marasmus than of any intestinal affection; and from this fact he concludes, that one of the offices of the bile is that of converting mucus, or the refuse of the chyle as it passes into the colon, into fat, which is absorbed and diffused over the system. I have already offered an objection to this theory (21).

76. When perfectly formed chyle, as that obtained from the thoracic duct, is chemically examined, it will

present a difference in composition, according to the nature
of the aliment from which it was elaborated. If the animal
has eaten substances of a fatty nature, the chyle will be
found milky white, a little heavier than distilled water,
with a strong and peculiar odour, and a saline and sensibly alkaline taste ; but if the food should not have contained fat, it will be opaline and almost transparent. Very
shortly after chyle is extracted from the living animal, it
becomes firm, and almost solid ; it then gradually sepa-
rates into three distinct parts ; the one solid, which remains
at the bottom of the vessel, the second liquid, and a third
that forms a very thin layer at the surface. The chyle at
the same time assumes a rose colour. Of the three parts
into which chyle thus spontaneously resolves itself, that
on the surface, of an opaque white, and which imparts
to the fluid the appearance of milk,* is a fatty body ; the
solid part, or coagulum, seems to be an intermediate substance between albumen and fibrin, for it unites several
properties which are common to the two ; it wants the
fibrous texture as well as the strength and elasticity of the
fibrin of the blood ; it is also more readily and completely
dissolved by caustic potass. The liquid part of chyle resembles the serum of the blood. The proportion, however,
of these several parts varies according to 'the nature of the
food.   There are species of chyle, such as that from
sugar, which contain very little *albuminous fibrin ;* others,
such as that from flesh, contain more. The fatty part
is very abundant where the food has contained grease
or oil, while there is scarcely any under other circumstances.

77. These observations are of great value to the physiologist, as well as to the pathologist, as they demonstrate

---

* The comparison which has been established between chyle and
milk has no real foundation ; for the former contains nothing which
agrees exactly with the constituents of the latter.

the fallacy of that proposition which has been so frequently advanced; viz. " that there are *many* species of food, but only *one* aliment;" intimating thereby, that all substances, by decomposition, contribute to form one identical, invariable, essentially nutritive principle, — the " *quod nutrit*" of ancient authors; whereas, nothing is more clear, than that the nature and composition of the chyle vary with each individual aliment.

78. Having explained all that is known with respect to the formation of chyle, we may next consider the manner in which it is absorbed and carried into the blood. The chyliferous vessels by which this office is performed have been already described (53). It is probable that the mesenteric glands, through which they pass, produce an important change on the chyle, but the nature of this change is wholly unknown : it is certain that these glands receive many blood-vessels, in proportion to their volume, and that they secrete a peculiar fluid, which may be extracted by compressing them between the fingers ; whence some physiologists have supposed, that they add a fluid to the chyle in order to purify it; while others, again, have contended, that their use is to produce a more intimate mixture of the elements which compose it. Much discussion has also arisen upon the existence of the *tact*, or sensibility of these vessels ; and although M. Majendie ridicules the supposition, there are not wanting facts to support the belief, that their mouths, like the pylorus, possess the power of discriminating between chyle and other less congenial fluids, which enables them to absorb the former, and to reject the latter ; and it is equally probable, that this selecting tact may be destroyed by disease, and that many evil consequences arise from it. The chyle is poured into the thoracic duct, together with the lymph which is brought hither from every part of the body by the lymphatic vessels, and thence carried into the subclavian vein, to be submitted to the action of the respiratory organs. It will,

therefore, be remembered, that a portion of the decayed and broken down materials is conveyed into the lungs, together with the new materials which are to repair the waste.

79. The nutritive principles of the aliment have now been traced, through all their changes, to the circulation. Let us then return to the excrementitious part which was left in the duodenum. This matter is pressed forward, by the peristaltic motion of the intestine, losing as it proceeds any portion of chyle which may have escaped the lacteals in the higher part of the small intestines, into the cæcum : its return being prevented by the valve already described (19), it accumulates to a certain extent in the colon, having now acquired that peculiar fœtor which distinguishes excrement : it is considerably retarded in this part of its passage by the cells or compartments into which this intestine is divided; at length, however, it enters the rectum, and, by forming a mass of considerable bulk, frequently distends its parietes, and thus creates a sensation of uneasiness, which announces the necessity of relief. If, however, this call be not imperious, and we neglect to obey it, the intestine becoming insensible to the stimulus of distension, the desire ceases, and may not recur for some time. This effect is greatly modified by the consistence of the fecal matter : if it be soft, or almost liquid, we shall be less able to resist its expulsion. The intervals at which this operation is performed will vary extremely in different individuals : some persons evacuate their fæces twice or thrice a day ; others, not more than once in two days ; and there are those who, although in perfect health, pass over a week or ten days without any evacuation. Habit also exerts a wonderful influence in regulating such periods : a person accustomed to the act at a certain hour of the day, will generally feel an inclination at the appointed season.

80. We have hitherto only considered the digestion of solid aliments; it now becomes necessary that we should

investigate the changes which fluids undergo, when introduced into the stomach. The subject teems with many curious physiological facts, and it is one of much importance to the pathologist, as it will enable him to appreciate the utility of liquid diet, and to understand the circumstances which should decide its preference.

81. It was long supposed, that liquids, like solids, passed through the pylorus into the small intestine, and were absorbed together with the chyle, or rejected with the excrement. It is not asserted that this never occurs ; but it is evident, beyond contradiction, that there exists another passage by which liquids can be conveyed to the circulation ; for it has been proved, that if a ligature be applied round the pyloric orifice, in such a manner as to obstruct the passage into the duodenum, the disappearance of the liquid from the cavity of the stomach is not so much as retarded. It is evident, therefore, that there must exist some other passage, although its nature and direction remain a matter of conjecture. I am strongly persuaded, that the *vena portæ* constitutes one of the avenues through which liquids enter the circulation ; and, in my Pharmacologia, I have expressed my belief,* and supported it by various arguments, that through this channel certain medicinal bodies find their way into the blood. In order to discover whether drinks are absorbed along with the chyle, M. Majendie made a dog swallow a certain quantity of diluted alcohol during the digestion of his food ; in half an hour afterwards, the chyle was extracted and examined : it exhibited no trace of spirit; but the blood exhaled a strong odour of it, and by distillation yielded a sensible quantity.

82. When liquids are introduced into the stomach, the changes which they undergo are determined by the nature of their composition.

83. When a liquid, holding nutritive matter in solu-

---

* Pharmacologia, edit. 6, vol. i. p. 127.

tion, is introduced into the stomach, it is either coagulated by the gastric juice, or its watery part is absorbed, and the solid matter deposited in the stomach; in both cases the product is afterwards chymified in the manner already described. Milk appears to be the only liquid aliment which nature has prepared for our nourishment; but it seems that she has, at the same time, provided an agent for rendering it solid; hence we may conclude that this form is an indispensable condition of bodies which are destined to undergo the processes of chymification and chylification; and that, unless some provision had existed for the removal of aqueous fluid from the stomach, the digestive functions could not have been properly performed. When the broth of meat is introduced into the stomach, the watery part is carried off, and the gelatine, albumen, and fat are then converted into chyme. Wine and fermented liquors undergo a similar change; the alcohol which they contain coagulates a portion of the gastric juices, and this residue, together with the extractive matter, gum, resin, and other principles which the liquid may contain, are then digested. Under certain circumstances, these liquids may observe a different law of decomposition, which will perhaps in some measure explain the different effects which such potations will produce : for example, the spirit may undergo a partial change in the stomach, and be even digested with the solid matter, or, on some occasions, converted into an acid by a fermentative process : this will be more likely to occur in vinous liquors, which contain ingredients favourable to the production of such a change; and hence the less permanent and mischievous effects of wines than of spirits.* The liquor termed *punch* will certainly, *cæteris paribus*, produce a less intoxicating effect than an equivalent quantity of spirit and water : this may be accounted for by supposing that

* See Pharmacologia, edit. 6. vol. ii. art. *Vinum.*

a portion of the alcohol is digested by the stomach into an acid, a process which is determined and accelerated by the presence of a fermentable acid like that of lemon, aided, perhaps, by the saccharine matter.

84. Oil, although possessed of the fluid form, does not appear to observe the law which governs the disposal of these bodies; it is not absorbed, but is entirely transformed into chyme in the stomach. To effect this, however, it seems essential that the stomach should be in a state of high energy, or it undergoes chemical decomposition, and becomes rancid ; nor will the stomach, unless it be educated to it, like those of some northern nations, digest any considerable quantity of it : and, since it cannot be absorbed, it must find its exit through the alimentary canal, and consequently prove laxative.

85. I have endeavoured to shew in the Pharmacologia, that certain salts are absorbed with the water which holds them in solution, unless they so far increase the peristaltic motion as to produce catharsis, in which case, they pass at once through the alimentary passage ; but should this not occur, they enter the circulation, and will sometimes exhibit their effects on distant organs. It is on this account that sulphate of magnesia proves diuretic in horses, for the bowels of these animals are not stimulated by that salt; and the same theory will explain why persons frequently experience an increase in their urine on drinking the weaker waters of Cheltenham.

86. It has been stated, that the chyle, together with the lymph, is poured into the sub-clavian vein. We know very little of the use of this latter fluid: it is conveyed by vessels, termed *lymphatics*, which appear to spring from extremely small roots in the substance of the membranes and of the cellular tissue, and in the parenchyma of the different organs. In man, these vessels uniformly traverse glands before they arrive at the venous system. The general opinion entertained upon the subject of lymphatic ab-

sorption, assigns to this order of vessels the office of returning the broken-down and useless parts of the various structures to the blood, in order that they may be finally ejected from the body. In examining the chemical composition of lymph, we find it to have a considerable analogy with the blood; which has induced M. Majendie to conclude that it is a part of that fluid, which, instead of returning to the heart by the veins, follows the course of the lymphatic vessels; for what object it is impossible even to offer a conjecture. He therefore doubts whether these vessels have any absorbing power, but endeavours to prove by experiments, which certainly have the merit of great plausibility, that the faculty of absorption is possessed by veins. Be this, however, as it may, it is certain, that the chyle, as well as those fluids which are absorbed from the stomach, are transmitted through the lungs for the purpose of undergoing such changes as may perfectly assimilate them with the blood. Every meal, therefore, must impose a certain labour upon these organs ; and it is probable, that the extent of this labour will vary with the nature of the food. It becomes, then, an object of the greatest pathological interest, to inquire into the relations which subsist between the functions of chylification and respiration, and to ascertain what species of food will require the greatest, what the least effort of the lungs to complete their sanguification. In cases of pulmonary disease, such a discovery would be of the highest value, in order that we may not impose upon an enfeebled organ more duty than is necessary for the preservation of life. Unfortunately, the facts which have been collected upon this subject are few, and even discordant. The faint light which science afforded us in the investigation of the preceding stages of digestion is here extinguished, and experience, embarrassed with a thousand sources of fallacy, is all that remains for us. Notwithstanding the numerous experiments which have been instituted, and the various

theories which have been formed, how extremely vague
and doubtful is our knowledge respecting the physiology
of respiration! It is true, that the chemist, by a refined
examination of the air, before and after it has been
respired, has ascertained that a quantity of oxygen is
absorbed, and replaced by an equivalent proportion of carbonic acid; but can any person accustomed to reflection
believe, that respiration serves no other purpose than that of
the removal of a certain portion of carbon from the blood?
A function which cannot be suspended for a minute
without the certain destruction of life, must surely have
some relation with the vital energy more intimate and important. The quantity of carbonic acid does not appear to
have that striking connexion with the quality or quantity
of our ingesta which our theory would have led to suppose.
Whoever will read an account of the results obtained by
Dr. Prout, in his examination of the "Quantity of carbonic acid gas emitted from the lungs during respiration, at different times, and under different circumstances,"* will retire from the perusal of the essay with
the mortifying conviction, that little or nothing is known
upon the subject: such, at least, was my conviction upon
that occasion. It must, however, teach us the folly of
hasty generalization, for nothing tends more to the perpe-
tuation of error. It has been well observed, that when we
have once tied up our ideas into bundles, the trouble, the
difficulty, the shame of untying them is felt even by superior minds. "*Sir,*" said Dr. Johnson, "*I don't like to
have any of my opinions attacked.—I have made up my
faggot, and if you draw out one, you weaken the whole.*"

87. If no material influence is produced upon the sum
of oxygen absorbed, or of carbonic acid disengaged, by the
different quantities and nature of our aliments, it follows,
that the conversion of chyle into blood is produced by
some other agent than that of the atmospheric air. At the

* Annals of Philosophy, vol. ii. p. 328.

same time, ample experience has taught us, that the nature
of our ingesta is not a matter of indifference to the
respiratory organs : diseased lungs are exasperated by
a certain diet, and pacified by one of an opposite kind.
The celebrated diver, Mr. Spalding, observed, that whenever he used a diet of animal food, or drank spirituous
liquors, he consumed in a much shorter period the oxygen
of the atmospheric air in his diving-bell; and he, therefore,
had learnt from experience to confine himself upon such
occasions to vegetable diet. He also found the same
effect to arise from the use of fermented liquors; and he
accordingly restricted himself to the potation of simple
water. The truth of these results is confirmed by the
habits of the Indian pearl-divers, who always abstain from
every alimentary stimulus previous to their descent into
the ocean. Those physicians who have witnessed the
ravages of pulmonary disease will readily concur in the
justness of these views. The experiments of Dr. Prout
would lead us to the conclusion, that less carbonic acid is
given off from the lungs during the influence of an alcoholic stimulant; but he justly observes, that this may
arise from its specific action upon the nerves : and, indeed,
it appears probable, that the evolution of carbon from the
blood is determined by nervous energy.* The principal
changes which the chyle undergoes during its passage
through the respiratory organs appear to consist in the
more perfect elaboration of some of its principles; for instance, the albumen is converted into fibrin, and the colouring matter acquires its more decided characteristics.
But these changes may be in a great measure produced

* The experiments of Drs. Prout and Fyfe have clearly shewn, that
whatever depresses the nervous energy, diminishes the quantity of carbonic acid expired. The depressing passions, violent and long-continued
exercise, low diet, mercurial irritation, and spirituous liquors, uniformly
produce this effect. The quantity is also, for the same reason, diminished
during sleep.

by the action of the pulmonary vessels. It has been estimated, that about eleven ounces of carbon and twenty
ounces of water are given off by the lungs during the
twenty-four hours; but what portion of these products are
to be placed to the account of the aliment has not been
ascertained. It does not even appear, that the useless carbon is always evolved from the blood during its passage
through these organs; it may be retained for want of sufficient nervous energy, and thus produce a morbid change
upon the body.

88. The quantity of pulmonary transpiration is also
influenced by various circumstances, especially the liquid
nature of the food, and the quantity of fluids taken into
the stomach. I have paid some attention to this circumstance, for it suggests many important links in the treatment of disease.*

89. The only safe conclusions at which we can arrive
upon this intricate subject, may be embodied in the following canons : *viz.* 1st, *That animal food proves more
stimulant to the lungs than vegetable aliment.* 2d, *That
fermented liquors are injurious to these organs, both on
account of their general effects upon the circulation, and
their specific action upon the nervous system ; increasing, on
the one hand, the necessity of respiratory changes, and on
the other, diminishing the energies of the organs by which
they are accomplished.* 3d, *That moderate exercise, hilarity
of mind, free ventilation, and abstinence from fermented
liquors, are essentially necessary in that stage of the digestive process at which the chyle is poured into the blood-
vessels, in order to promote the free evolution of carbonic
acid.*

90. The office of the kidneys in secreting urine may,
in reference to the present subject, be considered in a
double point of view ; as removing from the body, gene-

---

* See my Pharmacologia, vol. i. p. 192.

rally, certain principles whose presence must be noxious; and in carrying off some portion of the aliment which cannot be assimilated with the blood, or such useless products as may arise during the progress of its elaboration.   In examining the composition of urine, we shall find certain ingredients which existed in the blood, and which have therefore passed through the urinary organs without change; we shall, at the same time, discover peculiar compounds which owe their existence to the *acidifying* action of the kidneys upon certain substances contained in the blood. The principles derived from the blood by filtration are *water, lactic acid, with its accompanying animal matters,* the *fixed alkalies,* and *lime.*   The new compounds formed are *sulphuric* and *phosphoric acids,* from the sulphur and phosphorus in the blood ; *urea,* probably derived from albumen ; and *lithic acid.*   Dr. Prout observes, that in certain forms of disease the acidifying tendency of the kidneys is carried to an excess, and that *nitric acid, oxalic acid,* &c., are produced ; whereas, on the other hand, it is occasionally suspended, diminished, or altogether subverted ; and unchanged *albumen* or *blood,* neutral substances, as *sugar,* or even alkaline substances, as *ammonia,* &c., are separated in abundance ; while the *phosphorus* and *sulphur,* at the same time, pass without being acidified.

91. With respect to the character of the diseases attending these states of the urine, it will, says Dr. Prout, be generally found, that when acids are generated in excess, the urine is commonly small in quantity, and high-coloured, and the disease inflammatory ; when neutral or alkaline substances, the urine, on the contrary, is generally pale-coloured, and larger in quantity, and the diseases are those of irritation and debility.   In examining, however, the state of the urine, with reference to its pathognomonic indications, we must carefully distinguish between that which is voided after abstinence, and which is termed *urina potus,* and that which is voided five or six hours after

a meal, and which is distinguished by the appellation of *urina sanguinis*. The temperature and hygrometric state of the atmosphere ought also to be taken into consideration; for these circumstances, by modifying the quantity of water given off by the skin, will exert a considerable influence upon the urinary secretion. Nothing, however, produces a greater effect upon the character of the urine than the state of the digestive functions; and by carefully inspecting its appearances, many valuable indications may be obtained. It is true, that the practice of examining the urine has fallen into discredit, from the abuse which it has suffered in the hands of empiricism and imposture; * but the new views which modern chemistry has unfolded, and the valuable practical purposes to which they have been made subservient by the labours of Wollaston, Marcet, and Prout, ought to restore it to its merited reputation.

92. I shall conclude these remarks by stating, that one of the objects of the urinary secretion appears to be the removal of a portion of nitrogen, and perhaps also of oxygen, from the blood, as that of respiration is the abstraction of carbon. This hypothesis is supported by the ultimate analysis of lithic acid and urea. It is, at least, evident, that some principle is withdrawn from the circulation, whose presence would act upon the system as a destructive poison: total suppression of urine is followed in a few hours by insensibility; but this consequence is prevented by the discharge of a few drops only of the secretion.

93. The function of the skin may be considered as the

* The vulgar have ever considered the urine as a glass, in which the physician may behold every thing that passes within the body; and the quacks have, for obvious reasons, been willing to indulge the credulity. It has been stated, that the origin of the imposition of *urine casting* is to be looked for in the ignorance and barbarism of the middle ages, when the greater part of physicians were ecclesiastics, who either saw their patients in their churches, or were satisfied with inspecting their urine.

last link in the chain of the digestive process. It removes from the blood a considerable portion of water, with some saline matter; and in this respect it may be compared to the office of the kidneys, although, unlike them, its function may be suspended without immediately fatal consequences. ⸰Experiments have also proved that an acid is discharged by the cutaneous emunctories; and if this be suppressed, it appears to pass off by the kidneys, and to give origin to a deposit to be hereafter noticed.

94. From a review of all the transformations which the aliment undergoes, from its conversion into chyme to that into blood, can we arrange the different changes under distinct heads, so as to bring each under the operation of any general law? I fear that our present state of chemical knowledge will not afford a satisfactory solution of this problem. The production of chyle in the duodenum certainly differs in its nature from that of any of the secreted fluids, since the mass from which it is evolved is acted upon by foreign re-agents, as the bile and pancreatic liquor; whereas a secreted fluid is at once separated from the blood without the aid of any precipitant. In this point of view, the operation bears a closer analogy to a chemical process; but here the comparison must end, for we are unable to account for the presence of any of the new compounds by an analysis of the ingredients from which they are produced. If we admit the operation of a galvanic power, generated by the nerves, and directed through their means to the decomposition of the alimentary materials, and to their recombination into other forms, we shall obtain, if not a satisfactory solution of the problem, at least some clue for its investigation. We shall thus perceive, that elements having a strong chemical affinity for each other may be separated and reunited in different proportions; and we shall be able to explain why substances, distinguished by their strong attractions for each other, do not combine in the alimentary organs, as they

would in the vessels of our laboratory. But it will be asked, what reason there is for believing in the existence of any power analogous in its operation to electricity? This question cannot be better answered than by a relation of the ingenious experiments of Dr. Wilson Philip, who has clearly shewn that when a nerve is divided, so as entirely to intercept the transmission of its energy, its function may, to a certain degree, be supplied by an electrical stream from the galvanic battery. The eight pair of nerves were divided in the necks of three recently-fed rabbits, and every precaution was taken to keep their divided ends asunder. One of these animals, when subjected to the galvanic influence, remained singularly quiet, breathing freely, and with no more apparent distress than the twitches usually produced by electric action, which was in this case kept up without interruption. The other rabbits laboured strongly in their respiration. They were all three killed at the same period, and their stomachs successively opened. In the two non-galvanised animals chymification had scarcely made any progress; but in that which had been galvanised, the process appeared to have been completed.

95. It is not my intention, in this work, to enter into any speculations with respect to the more minute changes which may be supposed to take place under this galvanic influence of the nerves. My determination in this respect has been made, in consequence of learning from Dr. Prout that he has been long engaged in the investigation, and has arrived at some very curious and important results, which it is his intention shortly to give to the public. In the next place, such details would be wholly inconsistent with the practical objects of my present publication. I shall therefore conclude this part of my subject by observing, that most of the digestive products are acid; the chyme is uniformly distinguished by this character; and, if the experiments of Dr. Prout be correct, muriatic acid is

always present in the stomach: we may, therefore, suppose
that the nerves of this organ have the power of decomposing
the muriatic salts, and transferring its alkali to some
distant reservoir, perhaps the liver. The intestinal juices
are also acid; the fæces, unless they have undergone a
degree of putrefactive decomposition, redden litmus; the
urine, as well as the perspirable matter, are likewise acid;
and it is scarcely necessary to observe, that the only product of the respiratory function is carbonic *acid*.

96. If the nerves act like galvanic conductors, we may
explain the transferrence of matter from one organ to another, without the necessity of supposing the existence of
tubes or hollow vessels. Is it possible—I merely put it as
a query—that certain liquids may thus find their way from
the stomach to the kidneys?

RELATIONS OF THE DIGESTIVE FUNCTIONS WITH OUR SENSATIONS.

HUNGER:—*Theories to explain the Sensation.—Referred by the Author to a peculiar Condition of the Nerves.—Destroyed by Narcotics.—Practice of the Indians to counteract its cravings.—Its connexion with the state of the Stomach only secondary.—Chymification, Chylification, and Sanguification, may be considered as incompatible with each other.—Why an Interruption during a Meal destroys the Appetite.—The quality and not the quantity of Food produces Satiety.—Thirst:—Its final Causes.—Its proximate Cause.—General Phenomena of Inanition.—Sanguification attended by a desire of activity.—Of Exercise immediately before and after Meals.*

HUNGER.

97. WHEN the stomach is in a healthy condition, and has remained for some time empty, the well-known sensation of hunger is produced; to account for which, various hypotheses have been devised. Some have attributed its origin to the friction of the sides of the stomach upon each other, or to the dragging of the liver upon the diaphragm; others to the action of bile or acid vapours upon the stomach; to the compression of the nerves, or to the fatigue of the contracted fibres of the stomach: but such theories are subverted by the fact, that the stomach may remain empty for a long interval, during disease, without any sensation of hunger; and that when present, it may cease or be allayed by various causes, although food should not have been taken; as often happens after the accustomed period of repast is over, or from the sudden communication of news that over-

whelms us with grief or disappointment. The physiologists of the present day attribute the phenomenon to the stimulant action of the gastric juice upon the nerves of the stomach; and to support this opinion, Dr. Wilson Philip relates the following experiment. A person in good health was prevailed upon to abstain from eating for more than twenty-four hours, and during that interval to increase the appetite by more than ordinary exercise. At the end of this time he was extremely hungry; but, instead of eating, he excited vomiting by drinking warm water, and irritating the fauces. The water returned mixed only with a ropy fluid, such as the gastric juice is described to be. After this operation, not only all desire to eat was removed, but a degree of disgust was excited by seeing others eat. He, however, was prevailed upon to take a little bread and milk, which in a very short time ran into the acetous fermentation, as indicated by flatulence and acid eructation. I do not mean to deny that the presence of a portion of gastric juice may not contribute to the sensation of hunger; but I feel more disposed to refer the phenomenon to an energetic state of the gastric nerves, occasioned by an interval of inactivity, during which their vital powers may be supposed to accumulate. With respect to the actual quantity of gastric fluid in an empty stomach, we know little or nothing. It seems probable that it is supplied during digestion, and that its secretion corresponds with the nature and quantity of the ingesta. If a narcotic be applied to the nerves, their power is paralysed, and the sensation of hunger ceases; such an effect is produced by the juice of tobacco, although by long habit the stomach may become indifferent to its operation. Whenever the Indians of Asia and America undertake a long journey, and are likely to be destitute of provisions, they mix the juice of tobacco with powdered shells, in the form of small balls, which they retain in their mouths, the gradual solution of which serves to counteract the uneasy craving of the stomach. In like manner we may explain the operation of spirit in taking away the appetite of those who are not accustomed to it; while those who indulge the habit receive its stimulant without its narcotic impression.

98. Natural appetite, which is only the first degree of hunger, never appears to recur until the aliment previously introduced has been duly assimilated. It cannot, therefore, strictly speaking, be said to have an immediate reference to the state of the stomach; for although all the chyme may have long since passed out of that organ, if any delay occurs in its ulterior changes, appetite will not return, for the nervous energy is engaged in their completion, and cannot therefore accumulate in the stomach: on the contrary, in certain diseases, as in *tabes mesenterica*, notwithstanding the presence of alimentary matter in the stomach, the appetite is never pacified, in consequence, probably, of the diminished expenditure of vital power which attends the act of chylification in such cases, where only a small quantity of chyle is absorbed by the lacteals, and poured into the circulation. Voracity, or canine appetite, may sometimes depend upon a morbid state of the pylorus, which suffers the food to pass out of the stomach before it is properly chymified : such cases are attended with extreme emaciation. From these views we may deduce the following important corollary,—*that the several processes by which aliment is converted into blood cannot be simultaneously performed, without such an increased expenditure of vital energy as weak persons cannot, without inconvenience, sustain :* thus, chylification would appear to require the quiescence of the stomach, and sanguification to be still more incompatible with the act of chymification. If, therefore, the stomach be set to work during the latter stages of digestion, the processes will in weak persons be much disturbed, if not entirely suspended. Certain circumstances cause hunger to return at nearer intervals, by

accelerating the nutritive process; while others, by producing an opposite tendency, lengthen such intervals.

99. It is a well-known fact, that if a person be interrupted in his meal for a quarter of an hour, he finds, on resuming it, that his appetite is gone, although he may have not eaten half the quantity which he required. Dr. Wilson Philip explains this circumstance by supposing, that the gastric fluid which had accumulated has had time to combine with, and be neutralised by, the food he had taken; but those who believe with me, that a new supply of gastric fluid is furnished on the contact of every fresh portion of food, must seek for some other explanation. Will not the views which I have offered in the preceding paragraph afford a solution of the problem? viz. that during the suspension of the meal the food had entered upon its ulterior changes, and that the energies of the stomach had therefore declined.

100. The subsidence of appetite, or the feeling of satiety, is not produced by the *quantity*, but the *quality* of the food,—the very reverse of what would happen were the mere volume of the aliment alone necessary to pacify the cravings of the stomach. This is remarkably displayed in the habits of ruminating animals; for in wet and gloomy seasons, when the grass contains a diminished portion of nutritive matter, these animals are never satisfied—they are constantly in the act of grazing; whereas, in hot and dry weather, they consume the greater portion of their time in that of ruminating, or chewing the cud. I apprehend that this is not to be explained, as M. Majendie believes, to the sensibility of the mucous membrane of the stomach, but is to be solely referred to the fact, that the vital energy is only expended in decomposing such substances as are capable of furnishing chyle. Volume or bulk, however, is a necessary condition of wholesome food: the capacity of our digestive organs sufficiently proves that nature never intended them for the reception of highly

concentrated food. I some years ago directed considerable attention, in conjunction with some well-known agriculturists, to the nutritive value of different crops, as the food of cattle, and I constructed a logometric scale for the solution of various problems connected with the subject; but I soon found that mere *bulk* produced a very important influence, and that, to render one species of nutriment equivalent in its value to another, it was necessary to take into consideration the quantity of inert matter which furnished excrement.

THIRST.

101. This instinctive feeling announces to the individual the necessity of introducing a certain quantity of liquid into the system, in order to repair the waste which the body has sustained in the exercise of its functions; or to impart a due degree of solubility to the aliments which have been taken. We accordingly find that excessive perspiration increases the demand, and dry food is followed by the same effect. With the history of morbid thirst we have at present nothing to do. The sensation of thirst appears to reside in the throat and fauces, as that of hunger does in the stomach; and yet the intensity of this feeling does not bear any relation to the dryness of these parts; for in some cases where the tongue, to its very root, is covered with a thick and dry crust, there is little thirst; while, on the other hand, it is frequently intolerable at the very time the mouth is surcharged with a preternatural quantity of saliva: like hunger, I apprehend it must be referred to a particular condition of the nerves. The desire for drink after long speaking is analogous to thirst, but must not be confounded with it. The influence of salted food in exciting this sensation is not well understood.

102. Thirst is certainly under the control of habit:

those who indulge in the vicious habit of frequent potations are rendered thirsty by its privation. There are
some persons who have never experienced the sensation,
and who only drink from a sort of sympathy, but who
could live a long time without thinking of it, or without
suffering from the want of it. I have a lady, of fifty
years of age, at this time under my care, who has declared
that she is perfectly unacquainted with the nature of the
sensation. Sauvage relates two similar instances that
occurred to himself; and Blumenbach, also, quotes several examples of the same idiosyncrasy.

103. The sensations of hunger and thirst appear to be
incompatible with each other: when the stomach requires
food, there is no inclination to drink; and when thirst
rages, the very idea of solid aliment disgusts us. So,
again, those circumstances which tend to destroy appetite
may even excite thirst, such as the passions of the
mind, &c.

104. When the healthy system is in a condition to require food, besides the local sensation of hunger, there are
certain general phenomena which deserve notice; — a universal lassitude of the body is experienced; there is also a
sensation of pressure, or drawing down, in the epigastric
region; the diameter of the intestines becomes diminished,
and their peristaltic motion being at the same time increased, portions of contained air are successively dis-
placed, which give rise to gurgling sounds. There is, besides, an alteration in the situation of some of the abdominal viscera; they are less capable of sustaining pressure,
and they receive a less quantity of blood. M. Majendie
also supposes, that when the stomach is empty, all the
reservoirs contained in the abdomen are more easily distended by the matters which remain some time in them;
and he believes that this is the principal reason why bile
then accumulates in the gall-bladder. As soon as a certain quantity of food has entered the stomach, the general

feeling of lassitude gives place to that of renewed force, and this usually occurs more rapidly after the ingestion of liquid than of solid aliment; which is sufficient to prove that the phenomenon results from a local action upon the nerves of the stomach, since in neither case is it possible to suppose that any nutritive principle can have been so rapidly transferred to the system.

105. As soon as digestion commences, the blood flows with increased force to the organs destined for its completion; whence, in delicate persons, the operation is frequently attended with a diminution in the power of the senses, and a slight shiver is even experienced; the skin becomes contracted, and the insensible perspiration is diminished. As the process, however, proceeds, a reaction takes place; and, after it is completed, the perspiration becomes free, and often abundant. When the chyle enters the blood, the body becomes enlivened, and the stomach and small intestines having been liberated from their burden, oppose no obstacle to the free indulgence of that desire for activity, which nature has thus instinctively excited for our benefit. Then it is that animals are roused from that repose into which they had subsided during the earlier stages of digestion, and betake themselves to action; then it is that civilised man feels an aptness for exertion, although he mistakes the nature and object of the impulse, and, as Dr. Prout justly observes, is inclined to regard it as nothing more than a healthy sensation by which he is summoned to that occupation to which inclination or duty may prompt him. Thus, instead of being *bodily* active, the studious man receives it as a summons to *mental* exertion; the indolent man, perhaps, merely to *sit up and enjoy himself:* the libertine to commence his libations; and the votary of fashion to attend the crowded circles of gaiety and dissipation : in short, this feeling of renovated energy is used, or abused, in a thousand ways by different individuals,

without their ever dreaming that *bodily exercise, and that
alone,* is implied by it. The result of which is, that imperfect assimilation, and all its train of consequences, take
place.

106. Some difference of opinion has existed with regard to the utility or mischief of exercise immediately after
eating; but in this question, as in most others of the like
nature, the truth will be found to lie between the extremes.
Those who, from confounding the effects of gentle with
those of exhausting exercise, maintain the necessity of rest
for the perfect performance of the digestive process, appeal
to the experiment of Sir Busick Harwood, the mere relation of which will be sufficient to negative the inference
which they would deduce from its result. The Downing
Professor took two pointers, equally hungry, and equally
well fed ; the one he suffered to lie quiet after his meal,
the other he kept for above two hours in constant exercise.
On returning home, he had them both killed. In the
stomach of the dog that had remained quiet and asleep,
all the food was found chymified; but in the stomach of
the other dog, the process of digestion had scarcely commenced. Exercise, let it be remembered, must be measured in relation to the strength and habits of the individual : we have daily experience to prove that the
husbandman may return to his daily labour, and the
schoolboy to his gambols, immediately after a frugal
meal, without inconvenience or injury ; but the same degree of exercise to a person of sedentary habits, or of weak
stamina, would probably arrest and subvert the whole
process of digestion. The influence of habit, in rendering
exercise salutary or injurious, is shewn in a variety of
instances: a person who would suffer from the slightest
exertion after dinner, will undertake a fatiguing labour after
breakfast, however solid and copious that meal may have
been. If we assent to the proposition of the Cambridge
Professor, we must in consistency acknowledge, that ex-

ercise, *before* a meal, is at least as injurious as he would lead us to suppose it is *after* a repast : for if the valetudinarian take his dinner in a state of fatigue, he will assuredly experience some impediment in its digestion ; but are we to argue that, on this account, exercise is neither to precede nor follow a meal ? We may as well, without farther discussion, subscribe to the opinion of Hieronymus Cardanus, who, insisting upon the advantages of perfect rest, observes, that *trees live longer than animals because they never stir from their places.*

PART II.

OF THE

MATERIA ALIMENTARIA.

PART II.

MATERIA ALIMENTARIA.

INTRODUCTION.

*Population depends upon the Quantity, not the Quality, of
Food.— Immunity from Disease, how connected with
Salubrity of Diet.— The Views of the Political Econo-
mist in direct Opposition with those of the Physician.—
Animal and Vegetable Diet.— Whether Nitrogen be an
essential Element of Food.— Classification of Aliments.
— Nutritive and Digestible not Synonymous Terms.—
Digestibility of Food influenced by its Mechanical Con-
dition.— Cookery; Boiling, Roasting, &c.— CONDI-
MENTS: Salt, Vinegar, Spices, &c.—DRINKS: Water,
Gruel, Barley-water, Tea, Coffee, &c. Broths.— Fer-
mented Liquors.—Different Species of Wine.—Beer, &c.*

107. THOSE bodies which have possessed life can alone
be strictly considered as affording aliment to animals; yet
there exist a certain number of inorganic substances, such
as water, common salt, lime, &c., which, although incapable by themselves of nourishing, appear, when admi
nistered in conjunction with the former, to contribute

essentially to nutrition. The consideration, therefore, of
the *Materia Alimentaria* necessarily embraces, not only
the SUBSTANTIVE agents above stated, but those which,
from their *modus operandi,* are entitled to the distinctive
appellation of alimentary ADJECTIVES. Under the former
division will be arranged all the varieties of animal and
vegetable food; under the latter, the class of condiments
will merit our attention.

108. The necessity of dietetic regulations has ever
been opposed by that popular and sweeping proposition,
— that *man is omnivorous;* that there scarcely exists a
species of animal or vegetable being that has not been
applied as food by some nation or horde, without inconvenience; that, while one race subsists on roots and fruits,
another lives, as exclusively, on raw flesh of the grossest
description; and another, again, on a mixed diet, partly
animal, and partly vegetable; and yet that all are equally
nourished, equally healthy, and equally competent to discharge the various duties which circumstances may have
imposed upon them. It would be vain to deny that the
Author of Nature has so constructed us and our organs
of digestion, as to enable us gradually to accommodate
ourselves to every species of aliment, without injury. By
the same train of reasoning, the quantity, as well as
the period of a repast, would appear as immaterial as
its quality. The Esquimaux, who feeds voraciously on
the walrus, is frequently, from the precarious nature
of its supply, deprived for days of his favourite meal; and
yet bodily disease neither follows repletion in the one
case nor privation in the other. Is it, then, immaterial
to our health whether we feast with Apicius or starve
with Epicurus? Such, doubtless, is the conclusion at
which those who disparage the utility of a regulated regimen are so anxious to arrive; but it becomes the duty of
a writer upon Dietetics to inquire how far such opinions
are founded in truth. In the first place, it may be ob-

served that the population of a country must always advance in proportion to the facility with which children can be supported. The fertility of the several ichthy-ophagous nations, as well as that of the inhabitants of our fishing towns, is to be thus explained, and is not to be attributed, as Montesquieu believed, to the peculiar nature of their diet. In accounting, therefore, for the populous-ness of a district, the *quantity*, and not the *quality*, of the food is to be principally considered. With respect to the general health and vigour of a population, we must be ex-tremely cautious how we attempt to connect the immunity from disease with peculiarity of diet. The robust and healthy will sustain a regimen which would prove destruc-tive to their less hardy brethren. An innutritious diet may thus contribute to the general health of a community at the expense of its weaker individuals; for, by weeding out the latter, the proportion of the former must be aug-mented. The same observation applies with equal force to the other *non-naturals*.* In this respect, then, the

* What numerous examples might be adduced in illustration of this subject! The troops of uncivilised countries compensate for their defi-ciency in discipline by superiority of animal strength; because the less robust are swept from the ranks by the hardships to which they are ex-posed. This fact has been generally acknowledged, although the expla-nation of it has been frequently erroneous: the regimen of the Spartans has been a common theme of discussion; and the exclamation of Pausa-nias, after the battle of Platea, will readily occur to the reader. But a Spartan regimen will not give vigour to those who are naturally weak; and yet the practitioners of modern times have not unfrequently acted upon such a belief. In examining the bills of mortality, with the view of ascertaining the numbers who have died at different ages, in successive years, it will appear that the number of deaths under two years of age, from the year 1728 to that of 1750, annually fluctuated between nine and ten thousand; and that, in the latter half of the last century, it was di-minished to six or seven thousand: while, since the commencement of the present century, the number has averaged under five thousand five hundred. This striking diminution of mortality among children seems imputable to the correction of that vulgar error which led nurses to expose children to

views of the political economist are in direct opposition
to those of the physician : the object of the one, is the pro-
motion of the general good of a community, while that of
the other, is the preservation of its more feeble individuals.

109. Whether nature originally intended that man
should feed on animal or vegetable substances has afforded
a fertile theme for discussion. It is not my intention to
follow the various authors who have attempted to prove
that animal food was not eaten before the deluge, but was
introduced in consequence of the deterioration which the
herbage sustained on that occasion. Such questions may
serve to exercise the ingenuity of the casuist, but they
present no interest to the physician. It is sufficiently evident from the structure of our teeth, and from the extent
of the alimentary canal being less than that of the vegetable eater, and greater than that of the carnivorous animal, that man is *omnivorous*, and capable of subsisting on
aliment of every description. Broussonet, however, is
inclined to believe that man is more herbivorous than carnivorous in his nature ; and, from the proportion which
the different teeth bear to each other, he even ventures to
conclude, that his mixed diet should consist of animal and
vegetable food in the proportion of 20 to 12. No rule,
however, of this nature can possibly be established ; we
have only to consider the different effects produced upon
the body by these two species of aliment, to perceive that
the circumstances of climate, season, exercise, habit, age,

cold, in order to " *harden* their constitutions." The political economist
may, perhaps, censure the modern physician, as Plato did Herodicus,
for teaching the infirm to regulate their exercise and diet in such a manner as to prolong their lives. If by care and good nursing the sickly infant
be carried through the first years of his life, he may possibly fall a victim
to the diseases of puberty ; and the same principle, therefore, which
explains the diminished number of early deaths will also explain the
increasing rates of those of maturer age, and the more frequent occurrence of pulmonary disease : but are the terrors of the spring to encourage the apathy of the nurserymen during the season of winter?

and individual peculiarity, must oppose such an attempt at generalisation.

110. As every description of food, whether derived from the animal or vegetable kingdom, is converted into blood, it may be inferred that the ultimate effect of all aliments must be virtually the same; and that the several species can only differ from each other in the quantity of nutriment they afford, in the comparative degree of stimulus they impart to the organs through which they pass, and in the proportion of vital energy they require for their assimilation. Were the degree of excitement which attends the digestion of a meal commensurate with the labour imposed upon the organs which perform it, less irritation and heat would attend the digestion of animal than of vegetable food; for in the one case the aliment already possesses a composition analogous to that of the structure which it is designed to supply, and requires little more than division and depuration; whereas, in the other, a complicated series of decompositions and recompositions must be effected before the matter can be animalised, or assimilated to the body. But the *digestive fever,* if we may be allowed the use of that expression, and the complexity of the alimentary changes, would appear, in every case, to bear an inverse relation to each other. This must depend upon the fact of animal food affording a more highly animalised chyle, or a greater proportion of that principle which is essentially nutritive, as well as upon the immediate stimulus which the alimentary nerves receive from its contact. In hot countries, therefore, or during the heats of summer, we are instinctively led to prefer vegetable food; and we accordingly find that the inhabitants of tropical climates select a diet of this description: the Bramins in India, and the people of the Canary Islands, Brazils, &c., live almost entirely on herbage, grains, and roots, while those of the north use little besides animal food. On account of the superior nutritive

power of animal matter, it is equally evident that the degree of bodily exertion, or exercise, sustained by an individual should not be overlooked in an attempt to adjust the proportion in which animal and vegetable food should be mixed. Persons of sedentary habits are oppressed, and ultimately become diseased, from the excess of nutriment which a full diet of animal food will occasion; such a condition, by some process not understood, is best corrected by acescent vegetables. It is well known that artisans and labourers, in the confined manufactories of large towns, suffer prodigiously in their health whenever a failure occurs in the crops of common fruits; this fact was remarkably striking in the years 1804 and 1805. Young children* and growing youths generally thrive upon a generous diet of animal food; the excess of nutritive matter is consumed in the development of the body, and, if properly digested, imparts strength without repletion. Adults and old persons comparatively require but a small proportion of aliment, unless the nutritive movement be accelerated by violent exercise and hard labour.

111. Those who advocate the exclusive value of animal food, and deny the utility of its admixture with vegetable matter, adduce in proof of their system the rude health and Herculean strength of our hardy ancestors. The British aborigines, when first visited by the Romans, certainly do not appear to have been conversant with the cultivation of the ground, and, according to the early writers, Cæsar, Strabo, Diodorus Siculus, and others, their principal subsistence was on flesh and milk; but before any valid conclusion can be deduced from this circumstance, the habits of the people must be compared with those of their descendants. The history of later times will furnish us with a satisfactory answer to those

---

* The aliment of almost every animal, in its first stage of life, is composed of animal matter; even graminivorous birds are nourished by the yolk for several days after being hatched.

who deny the necessity of vegetable aliment. We learn from the London bills, that scurvy raged to such an excess in the seventeenth century as to have occasioned a very great mortality : at this period the art of gardening had not long been introduced. It appears that the most common articles of the kitchen garden, such as cabbages, were not cultivated in England until the reign of Catharine of Arragon ; indeed, we are told that this queen could not procure a salad until a gardener was sent for from the Netherlands to raise it. Since the change thus, happily introduced into our diet, the ravages of the scurvy are unknown.

112. It follows, then, that in our climate a diet of animal food cannot, with safety, be exclusively employed. It is too highly stimulant ; the springs of life are urged on too fast; and disease necessarily follows. There may, nevertheless, exist certain states of the system which require such a preternatural stimulus; and the physician may, therefore, confine his patient to an animal regimen with as much propriety as he would prescribe opium, or any other remedy. By a parity of reasoning, the exclusive use of vegetable food may be shewn to be inconsistent with the acknowledged principles of dietetics, and to be incapable of conveying a nourishment sufficiently stimulating for the active exertions which belong to our present civilised condition. At the same time it must be allowed that an adherence to vegetable diet is usually productive of far less evil than that which follows the use of an exclusively animal regimen.

113. The science of chemistry had no sooner demonstrated that all the different tissues of the animal body contained azot (nitrogen), than it became a question amongst physiologists, whether that element were derived from the food introduced into our stomachs, or from the atmospheric air inhaled by our lungs ? To the practical physician this subject may not perhaps appear to pre-

sent any points of professional interest; but the experiments which have been lately instituted by M. Majendie, in support of the former opinions, have furnished results which, in my judgment, are susceptible of some useful applications to practice. M. Majendie observes, that the partisans of the theory he proposes to subvert insist particularly upon the example of the herbivorous animals, which are supported exclusively upon *non-azotised* matter; upon the history of certain people that live entirely upon rice and maize; upon that of negroes, who can live a long time without eating any thing but sugar; and, lastly, upon what is related of *caravans,* which, in traversing the deserts, have for a long time had only gum in place of every sort of food. Were it, says he, indeed proved by these facts that men can live a long time without *azotised* food, it would be necessary to acknowledge that azot has an origin different from the food; but the facts cited by no means sustain this proposition, for almost all the vegetables upon which man and animals feed contain more or less azot: for example, the impure sugar that the negroes eat presents a considerable proportion of it; and with regard to the people, as they say, who feed upon rice or maize, it is well known that they eat milk or cheese: now *cusein* is the most azotised of all the nutritive proximate principles. In order to acquire some more exact notions on this subject, M. Majendie submitted several animals, during a necessary period, to the use of food of which the chemical composition was accurately ascertained. I shall present the reader with an account of these experiments, and then explain the different, but not less important conclusions, which I deduce from their results. He took a small dog of three years old, fat, and in good health, and put it to feed upon sugar alone, and gave it distilled water to drink: it had as much as it chose of both. It appeared very well in this way of living for the first seven or eight days; it was brisk, active, eat eagerly, and drank in its usual manner. It began to get thin in the second week, although its appetite continued good, and it took about six or eight ounces of sugar in twenty-four hours. Its alvine excretions were neither frequent nor copious; that of the urine was very abundant. In the third week its leanness increased, its strength diminished, the animal lost its liveliness, and its appetite declined. At this period there was developed upon one eye, and then on the other, a small ulceration on the centre of the transparent cornea; it increased very quickly, and in a few days it was more than a line in diameter; its depth increased in the same proportion; the cornea was very soon entirely perforated, and the humours of the eye ran out. This singular phenomenon was accompanied with an abundant secretion of the glands of the eyelids. It, however, became weaker and weaker, and lost its strength; and, though the animal eat from three to four ounces of sugar per day, it became so weak that it could neither chew nor swallow; for the same reason every other motion was impossible. It expired the thirty-second day of the experiment. M. Majendie opened the animal with every suitable precaution. He found a total want of fat; the muscles were reduced to more than five-sixths of their ordinary size; the stomach and intestines were also much diminished in volume, and strongly contracted. The gall and urinary bladders were distended by their proper fluids, which M. Chevreul was called upon to examine. That distinguished chemist found in them nearly all the characters which belong to the urine and bile of *herbivorous* animals; that is, that the urine, instead of being acid, as it is in *carnivorous* animals, was sensibly alkaline, and did not present any trace of uric acid, nor of phosphate. The bile contained a considerable portion of *picromel;* a character considered as peculiar to the bile of the ox, and, in general, to that of herbivorous animals. The excrements were also examined by

M. Chevreul, and were found to contain very little azot, whereas they usually furnish a considerable quantity.

114. M. Majendie considered that such results required to be verified by new experiments : he accordingly repeated them on other dogs, but always with the same conclusions. He therefore considered it proved, that sugar, by itself, is incapable of supporting dogs. This want of the nutritive quality, however, might possibly be peculiar to sugar : he therefore proceeded to inquire, whether other substances, *non-azotised*, but generally considered as nutritive, would be attended with the same consequences. He fed two dogs with olive oil and distilled water, upon which they appeared to live well for about fifteen days ; but they afterwards underwent the same series of accidents, and died on the thirty-sixth day of the experiment. In these cases, however, the ulceration of the cornea did not occur.

115. Gum is another substance that does not contain azot, but which is considered as nutritive. To ascertain whether it acted like sugar and oil, he fed several dogs with this substance, and the phenomena which he observed did not differ sensibly from those above described.

116. The same distinguished physiologist lately repeated the experiment, by feeding a dog with butter, an animal substance free from azot. Like the other animals, it was supported by this food very well at first ; but, in about fifteen days, it began to lose flesh and to become weak : it died the thirty-sixth day, although, on the thirty-fourth day, he gave it as much flesh as it would eat, a considerable quantity of which it took for two days. The right eye of this animal presented the ulceration of the cornea that he noticed in those which were fed on sugar. The opening of the body presented the same modifications of the bile and urine. In order to make the evidence furnished by these experiments complete, after having given

to dogs separately, oil, gum, or sugar, he opened them, and ascertained that these substances were each reduced to a particular chyme in the stomach, and that they afterwards furnished an abundant chyle; whence he argues, that if these different substances are not nourishing, it cannot be attributed to the want of digestion.

117. Now, giving all due credit to the accuracy and good faith with which these experiments were performed, what do their results shew? That the azot of the organs is produced by the food, says M. Majendie, and consequently that no substance which does not contain this principle can support life. By no means: they merely prove that an animal cannot be supported by highly-concentrated aliment. In contradiction to the theory of Majendie, we know that sugar is highly nutritive, provided it be properly mixed with a quantity of substantial viands; it is certain that, in the process of making hay, if well performed, it will be found that the nutritive matter is greatly increased by the partial conversion of the cruder mucilaginous sap into a substance analogous to sugar; as we find that animals thrive faster with this food, and prefer it to that which is left on the ground, and found in a state of self-made hay. Horses fed on concentrated aliment are invariably liable to various diseases, originating from diseased action in the stomach, and hence arise broken wind, as it is termed, staggers, blindness, &c. The intolerable fetid odour of sulphuretted hydrogen gas, perceptible when post-horses are fed with oats and beans only, cannot have escaped observation; and it affords sufficient proof of the mischief which arises from a too-concentrated diet. The same remark applies to men; and I shall have occasion to shew hereafter, that the use of chocolate, butter, cream, sugar, and rich sauces, without a due admixture of bread, potatoes, and other less nutritive aliments, is invariably attended with disordered digestion. Unless the taste be

vitiated by habit, there exists an instinctive aversion to such food.

> ——————"The prudent taste
> Rejects, like bane, such loathsome lusciousness."

The Kamtschadales are frequently compelled to live on fish-oil, but they judiciously form it into a paste with saw-dust, or the rasped fibres of indigenous plants.

Of the Classification of Aliments.

118. The arrangements which different authors have proposed will be found to vary according to the particular theory by which each may have been influenced. The chemist investigates the composition of an aliment, and arranges it according to the proximate principles which predominate in its composition. The naturalist, on the other hand, merely considers to what division in his system each article of diet belongs, and assigns to it a corresponding place in his arrangement; while the empirical practitioner distributes the various kinds of food in an order which answers to his notions of their relative nutritive value, or to the supposed facility with which they are digested in the stomach. If there be any truth in our dietetic researches, or any natural affinity between the objects of our classification, the theory of the arrangement will be unimportant; for, however greatly the roads of our pursuit may vary, we must ultimately arrive at the same goal.

119. Chemistry has satisfactorily demonstrated the nature of these proximate principles of organic matter, upon the presence of which the nutritive qualities depend, viz. *fibrin, albumen, gelatin, oil and fat, gluten, fecula, or starch, mucilage, sugar, acids*, &c. Assuming that the variety, observable in the nutritive value of different sub-

stances arises from the predominance of one or more of such principles, we may conveniently distribute the Nu-TRIENTIA into the following nine classes :

Cl. I. Fibrinous Aliments. Comprehending the flesh and blood of various animals, especially such as have arrived at puberty : venison, beef, mutton, hare.

Cl. II. Albuminous. Eggs; certain animal matter.

Cl. III. Gelatinous Aliments. The flesh of young animals : veal, chickens, calf's foot, certain fishes,

Cl. IV. Fatty and Oily Aliments. Animal fats, oils, and butter; cocoa, &c.; ducks, pork, geese, eels, &c.

Cl. V. Caseous Aliments. The different kinds of milk, cheese, &c.

Cl. VI. Farinaceous Aliments. Wheat, barley, oats, rice, rye, potato ; sago, arrow-root, &c.

Cl. VII. Mucilaginous Aliments. Carrots, turnips, asparagus, cabbage, &c.

Cl. VIII. Sweet Aliments. The different kinds of sugar, figs, dates, &c.; carrots.

Cl. IX. Acidulous Aliments. Oranges, apples, and other acescent fruits.

To these we may add Condiments; such as salt, the varieties of pepper, mustard, horse-radish, vinegar, &c.

120. In classing the different species of potations, we may, in like manner, be governed by the chemical composition which distinguishes them. They may be arranged under four divisions, viz.

Cl. I. Water. Spring, river, well water, &c.

Cl. II. The Juices and Infusions of Vegetables and Animals. Whey, tea, coffee, &c.

Cl. III. Fermented Liquors. Wine, beer, &c.

Cl. IV. The Alcoholic Liquors, or Spirits. Alcohol, brandy, rum, &c.

121. Before we attempt to appreciate the value of the different substances arranged under the foregoing

classes, it will be necessary to caution the reader against
the popular error, of regarding the terms digestible and
nutritive as synonymous and convertible. A substance
may be highly nutritive, and yet be digested with difficulty; that is to say, it may require all the powers of the
digestive organs to convert it into chyle, and yet, when so
converted, it may afford a principle of highly-restorative
energy : this is the case with some of the fatty and oily
aliments.* On the contrary, there are substances which
apparently pass out of the stomach with sufficient readiness, but afford but little comparative support to the body.

122. Writers on dietetics have descanted very learn-
edly upon what they please to term the *perspirability*
and *alkalescency* of certain aliments. To the former I am
quite unable to attach any precise meaning ; with respect
to the latter, I apprehend that it is intended to express a
highly-nutritive quality, with a certain degree of indigestibility. *Heavy* and *light,* as applied to food, are terms
equally vague and indefinite, and ought never to be introduced into writings which aspire to the character of philosophical precision. The same observation may be extended
to the epithet *bilious* (74).

123. It is only necessary to reflect upon the chemical
and mechanical processes by which chymification is performed in the stomach (65), to perceive, that the digestibility of a substance may depend upon other circumstances
than that of its chemical composition. Its mechanical
state, with regard to texture and consistence, are of the
highest importance ; and if we attempt to deduce any law
upon this subject, from the known solubility of a substance
out of the body, we shall fall into several fatal errors. It
will be necessary to investigate this question with some
attention; for it not only explains the relative digestibility

---

* It has been calculated, that an ounce of fat meat affords nutriment
equal to four ounces of lean.

of aliments, but furnishes the only true basis for a system of skilful cookery.

124.   The healthy stomach disposes most readily and effectually of solid food, of a certain specific degree of density, which may be termed its *digestive texture;* if it exceed this, it will require a greater length of time, and more active powers, to complete its chymification; and if it approaches too nearly to a gelatinous condition, the stomach will be equally impeded in its operations.   It is, perhaps, not possible to appreciate or express the exact degree of firmness which will confer the highest order of digestibility upon food;* indeed, this zero may vary in different individuals; but we are taught by experience, that no meat is so digestible as tender mutton: when well conditioned, it appears to possess that degree of consistence which is most congenial to the stomach; and in this country it is perhaps more universally used than any other animal food.   Wedder mutton, or the flesh of the castrated animal, is in perfection at five years, and is by far the sweetest and most digestible.   Ewe mutton is best at two years' old.   Beef appears to be not so easy of digestion; its texture is firmer, but it is equally nutritive.   Much, however, will depend upon the period which has elapsed since the death of the animal, and more upon the method of cookery; in short, it would be worse than useless to attempt the construction of any scale to represent the nutritive and digestive qualities of the different species of food: the observations here introduced are merely noticed for the sake of illustrating those general principles whose application can alone afford us any rational theory of diet.

125.   It will not be difficult to understand why a certain texture and coherence of the aliment should confer

---

* Some experiments were instituted for this purpose by Gosse, of Geneva; but the conclusions deduced from them are by no means satisfactory.   He confounds solubility with digestibility, which in itself is sufficient to vitiate his reasoning.

upon it digestibility, or otherwise. Its conversion into chyme is effected by the solvent power of the gastric juice, aided by the *churning* which it undergoes by the motions of the stomach; and unless the substance introduced possess a suitable degree of firmness, it will not yield to such motions: this is the case with soups and other liquid aliments; in such cases, therefore, nature removes the watery part (83) before digestion can be carried forward. It is on this account that oils are digested with so much difficulty; and it is probable that jellies, and other glutinous matters, although containing the elements of nourishment in the highest state of concentration, are not digested without considerable difficulty; in the first place; on account of their evading the grappling powers of the stomach, and in the next, in consequence of their tenacity opposing the absorption of their more fluid parts. For these reasons I maintain, that the addition of isinglass, and other glutinous matter, to animal broths, with a view to render them more nutritive to invalids, is a pernicious custom.

126. The texture of animal food is greatly influenced by the age, sex, habits, condition, diet, and description of death of the animal which furnishes it. In proportion, generally, to the age, its flesh is coarser and more firm in texture, as every one must have noticed in eating birds. If the flesh of mutton and lamb, beef and veal, are compared, they will be found of a different texture, the two young meats are of a more stringy, indivisible nature than the others, which makes them harder of digestion. It has been also justly observed, that young animals differ from old ones in the distribution of the fat, which in the latter is chiefly collected in masses or layers, external to the muscles; whereas, in the former, it is more interspersed among the muscular fibres, giving the flesh a marbled appearance, which is always a desirable property of butcher's meat. The texture of food will also vary according to the

wild or domesticated state of the animal; that of the former is more dense, although highly nutritive. The sex also modifies the quality of the flesh, that of the female being always more delicate and finer-grained than that of the entire male, whose fibres are denser; the influence of the genital organs upon this occasion is very extraordinary; it is generally believed, that the flavour of the female is even improved by removing the ovaries, or *spaying* them, as it is called. Every day the testes are permitted to remain, even though totally inactive with regard to their proper function, injures the delicacy of the veal of the bull calf; and an animal which is not castrated until after puberty always retains much of the coarseness of the entire male. The mode of killing an animal has been considered, from the remotest ages, as capable of affecting the quality of its meat. The flesh of hunted animals is characterised by peculiar tenderness.; the same effect is produced by any lingering death. This fact probably explains the policy of those old municipal laws, which ordained that no butcher should offer or expose any bull-beef for sale, unless it had previously been baited; and it is upon the same principle only, that the quality of pig's flesh could be improved by the horrid cruelty of whipping them to death, as said to be practised by the Germans. The action of vinegar, administered to an animal some hours before killing it, is also known to be capable of rendering its flesh less tough. It is a common practice in the country to give a spoonful of this acid to poultry, when they are intended for the immediate service of the table.

127. Nothing, however, tends more effectually to ameliorate the rigidity of the animal fibre, than incipient putrefaction. The length of time that meat ought to be kept after it is killed will necessarily depend upon its tendency to undergo the putrid fermentation, and the prevalence of those circumstances which are inclined to favour it.

128. The circumstances which have been just enumerated, as being capable of influencing the texture of our food, and consequently its degree of digestibility, are, however, unimportant when compared with the modifying powers of cookery, which I shall now proceed to examine.

129. By cookery, alimentary substances undergo a twofold change; their principles are *chemically* modified, and their textures *mechanically* changed. The extent and nature, however, of these changes will greatly depend upon the manner in which heat has been applied to them; and if we inquire into the culinary history of different countries, we shall trace its connexion with the fuel most accessible to them. This fact readily explains the prevalence of the peculiar species of cookery which distinguishes the French table, and which has no reference, as some have imagined, to the dietetic theory, or superior refinement,.of the inhabitants.

130. BOILING. By this operation, the principles not properly soluble are rendered softer, more pulpy, and, consequently, easier of digestion; but the meat, at the same time, is deprived of some of its nutritive properties by the removal of a portion of its soluble constituents: the albumen and gelatin are also acted upon; the former being solidified, and the latter converted into a gelatinous substance. If, therefore, our meat be boiled too long or too fast, we shall obtain, where the albumen predominates, as in beef, a hard and indigestible mass, like an overboiled egg; or, where the gelatin predominates, as in young meats, such as veal, a gelatinous substance equally injurious to the digestive organs. Young and viscid food, therefore, as veal, chickens, &c., are more wholesome when roasted than when boiled, and are easier digested. Dr. Prout has very justly remarked, that the boiling temperature is too high for a great many of the processes of cooking, and that a lower temperature and a greater time, or a *species of infusion*, are better adapted for most of them.

This is notorious with substances intended to be *stewed*, which, even in cookery books, are directed to be *boiled slowly* (that is, not at all), and for a considerable time. The ignorance and prejudice existing on these points is very great, and combated with difficulty ; yet, when we take into account their importance, and how intimately they are connected with health, they will be found to deserve no small share of our attention.* The loss occasioned by boiling partly depends upon the melting of the fat, but chiefly from the solution of the gelatine and osmazone : mutton generally loses about one-fifth, and beef about one-fourth, of its original weight. Boiling is particularly applicable to vegetables, rendering them more soluble in the stomach, and depriving them of a considerable quantity of *air*, so injurious to weak stomachs. But, even in this case, the operation may be carried to an injurious extent; thus, potatoes are frequently boiled to the state of a dry, insipid powder, instead of being preserved in that state in which the parts of which they are composed are rendered soft and gelatinous, so as to retain their shape, yet be very easily separated. On the other hand, the cabbage tribe, and carrots, are frequently not boiled long enough, in which state they are highly indigestible. In conducting this process, it is necessary to pay some attention to the quality of the water employed ; thus, mutton boiled in hard water is more tender and juicy than when soft water is used ; while vegetables, on the contrary, are rendered harder and less digestible when boiled in hard water.

131. Roasting. By this process the fibrine is corrugated, the albumen coagulated, the fat liquefied, and the water evaporated. As the operation proceeds, the surface becomes first brown, and then scorched; and the ten-

---

* Hence it is, that beef tea and mutton tea are much more calculated for invalids than the broths of these meats.

dinous parts are rendered softer and gluey. Care should
always be taken that the meat should not be *over-done,* nor
ought it to be *under-dressed;* for although in such a state
it may contain more nutriment, yet it will be less digestible, on account of the density of its texture. This fact has
been satisfactorily proved by the experiments of Spallanzani;* and Mr. Hunter † observes, that *" boiled,* and
roasted, and even *putrid* meat, is easier of digestion than
raw." Animal matter loses more by roasting than by
boiling : it has been stated above, that by this latter process mutton loses one-fifth, and beef one-fourth; but by
roasting, these meats lose about one-third of their weight.
In roasting, the loss arises from the melting out of the fat,
and the evaporating of the water; but the nutritious matter
remains condensed in the cooked solid ; whereas, in boiling, the gelatine is partly abstracted. Roast are, therefore,
more nutritive than boiled meats. ‡

132. FRYING. This process is, perhaps, the most
objectionable of all the culinary operations. The heat is
applied through the medium of boiling oil, or fat, which
is rendered empyreumatic, and therefore extremely liable
to disagree with the stomach.

133. BROILING. By this operation, the sudden
browning or hardening of the surface prevents the evaporation of the juices of the meat, which imparts a peculiar
tenderness to it. It is the form selected, as the most
eligible, by those who seek to invigorate themselves by
the art of *training.*

134. BAKING. The peculiarity of this process depends upon the substance being heated in a confined
space, which does not permit the escape of the fumes

* Spallanzani on Digestion, vol. i. p. 277.

† Hunter on the Animal Economy, p. 220.

‡ It has been computed that, from the dissipation of the nutritive
juices by boiling, one pound of *roasted* contains as much nourishment as
two of boiled meat.

arising from it; the meat is, therefore, from the retention of its juices, rendered more sapid and tender. But baked meats are not so easily digested, on account of the greater retention of their oils, which are, moreover, in an empyreumatic state. Such dishes accordingly require the stimulus of various condiments to increase the digestive powers of the stomach.

OF CONDIMENTS.

135. These may be defined substances which are, in themselves, incapable of nourishing, but which, in concert with our food, promote its digestion, or correct some of its deleterious properties. The existence and necessity of such agents are far more universal and important than has been generally supposed.* The bitter principle which exists in the composition of grasses and other plants appears to be essential to the digestion of herbivorous animals; it acts as a natural stimulant; for it has been shewn, by a variety of experiments, that it passes through the body without suffering any diminution in its quantity, or change in its nature. No cattle will thrive upon grasses which do not contain a portion of this vegetable principle: this fact has been most satisfactorily proved by the researches of Mr. Sinclair, gardener to the Duke of Bedford, which are recorded in that magnificent work, the " *Hortus Gramineus Woburnensis.*" They shew, that if sheep are fed on yellow turnips, which contain little or no bitter principle, they instinctively seek for, and greedily devour, any provender which may contain it; and that if they cannot so obtain it, they become diseased and die. We are ourselves conscious of the invigorating effects of slight bitters upon our stomach; and their presence in malt liquors not only tends to diminish the noxious effects of such potations, by counteracting the indirect debility

* See my PHARMACOLOGIA, edition 6th, vol. i. p. 145.

which they are liable to occasion, but even to render them, when taken in moderation, promoters of digestion. The custom of infusing bitter herbs in vinous drinks is very ancient and universal. The *poculum absinthiatum* was regarded in remote ages as a wholesome beverage, and the wormwood was, moreover, supposed to act as an antidote against intoxication. Civilisation has, in a great measure, destroyed our natural taste for bitters; while, by improving our food, it has probably rendered its stimulus less necessary. The Swiss peasant cheers himself amid the frigid solitude of his glaciers with a spirit distilled from *gentian,* the extreme bitterness of which is relished with a glee that is quite unintelligible to a more cultivated taste. It may be safely affirmed, that the utility of this condiment is in an inverse ratio with the nutritive, or rather digestible power of a vegetable substance; and we accordingly find, in conformity with that universal scheme of self-adjustment and compensation, so visible in all the operations of nature, that cultivation, which exalts and extends the nutritive powers of vegetable bodies, generally diminishes their bitterness in the same proportion. The natural history of the potato, already alluded to (4), offers a good illustration of this fact.

136. From the different nature of condiment, it has been usually divided into three classes; viz. the *saline,* the *spicy* or *aromatic,* and the *oily.*

137. SALT appears to be a necessary and universal stimulus to animated beings; and its effects upon the vegetable as well as animal kingdom have furnished objects of the most interesting inquiry to the physiologist, the chemist, the physician, and the agriculturist. It appears to be a natural stimulant to the digestive organs of all warm-blooded animals, and that they are instinctively led to immense distances in pursuit of it. This is strikingly exemplified in the avidity with which animals in a wild state seek the salt pans of Africa and America, and in the

difficulties they will encounter to reach them : this cannot
arise from accident or caprice, but from a powerful instinct,
which, beyond control, compels them to seek, at all risks,
that which is salubrious. To those who are anxious to
gain further information upon this curious subject, I would
recommend the perusal of a work entitled " *Thoughts on
the Laws relating to Salt, by Samuel Parkes, Esq.*," and
a small volume by my late lamented friend, Sir Thomas
Bernard, on the " *Case of the Salt Duties, with Proofs
and Illustrations.*" We are all sensible of the effect of
salt on the human body ; we know how unpalatable
fresh meat and vegetables are without it.   During the
course of my professional practice, I have had frequent
opportunities of witnessing the evils which have attended
an abstinence from salt. In my examination before a
committee of the House of Commons in 1818, appointed for
the purpose of inquiring into the laws respecting the salt
duties, I stated, from my own experience, the bad effects
of a diet of unsalted fish, and the injury which the poorer
classes, in many districts, sustained in their health from
an inability to procure this essential condiment. I had
some years ago a gentleman of rank and fortune under my
care, for a deranged state of the digestive organs, accompanied with extreme emaciation. I found that, from some
cause which he could not explain, he had never eaten any
salt with his meals : I enforced the necessity of his taking
it in moderate quantities, and the recovery of his digestive
powers was soon evinced in the increase of his strength
and condition. One of the ill effects produced by an
unsalted diet is the generation of worms. Mr. Marshall
has published the case of a lady who had a natural anti-
pathy to salt, and was in consequence most dreadfully
infested with worms during the whole of her life. (*London
Medical and Physical Journal*, vol. xxix. No. 231.) In
Ireland, where, from the bad quality of the food, the
lower classes are greatly infested with worms, a draught

of salt and water is a popular and efficacious anthelmintic.
Lord Somerville, in his Address to the Board of Agriculture,
gave an interesting account of the effects of a punishment
which formerly existed in Holland. " The ancient laws
of the country ordained men to be kept on bread alone,
UNMIXED WITH SALT, as the severest punishment that
could be inflicted upon them in their moist climate. The
effect was horrible; these wretched criminals are said to
have been devoured by worms engendered in their own
stomachs." The wholesomeness and digestibility of our
bread are undoubtedly much promoted by the addition of
salt which it so universally receives.*

138. If the utility of salt be thus established, it may
be asked, how it can happen that salted provisions should
ever produce those diseases which experience has shewn
to arise from their use ? It is true that a certain proportion
of this condiment is not only useful but indispensable; but
an excess of it is as injurious as its moderate application is
salutary. This observation applies with as much force to
the vegetable as to the animal kingdom; a small proportion
applied as a manure, promotes vegetation in a very remarkable manner; whereas a larger quantity actually destroys
it. The experiments of Sir John Pringle have also shewn,
that a little salt will accelerate putrefaction, and a large
quantity prevent it. In explaining the operation of *salting*
meat, and in appreciating the effects of such meat as food,
it will be necessary to advert to a chemical fact which has
not hitherto attracted the attention which its importance
merits. The salt thus combined with the animal fibre
ought no longer to be considered as the condiment upon
which so much has been said; a chemical combination
has taken place, and, although it is difficult to explain the
nature of the affinities which have been brought into action,

* A pound of salt is generally added to each bushel of flour. Hence
it may be presumed, that every adult consumes two ounces of salt per
week, or six pounds and a half per annum, in bread only.

or that of the compound to which they have given origin, it is sufficiently evident that the texture of the fibre is so changed as to be less nutritive, as well as less digestible. If we are called upon to produce any chemical evidence in support of such an assertion, we need only relate the experiment of M. Eller, who found, that if salt and water be boiled in a copper vessel, the solution will contain a notable quantity of that metal; whereas, if, instead of heating a simple solution, the salt be previously mixed with beef, bacon, or fish, the fluid resulting from it will not contain an atom of copper. Does not this prove that the process of salting meat is something more than the mere saturation of the animal fibre with muriate of soda?

139. The beneficial operation of salt as a condiment is proved by ample experience : theory has had no share in establishing the fact; and, in the present state of our physiological knowledge, it will be, perhaps, difficult to offer a theory for its explanation. It may probably only operate as a stimulant upon the alimentary passages, although to those who are disposed to place any confidence in the views of Dr. Prout (95), an hypothesis will necessarily suggest itself, which, on the present occasion, it is not my intention either to support or invalidate. The subject is in good hands; and I look forward with some degree of impatience for the result of more extended researches.

140. VINEGAR. This acid, in small quantities, is a grateful and wholesome stimulant; it will often check the chemical fermentation of certain substances in the stomach, and prevent vegetable matter in its raw state from inducing flatulence; but its use requires caution, and in some morbid states of the system it is obviously improper. Fatty and gelatinous substances frequently appear to be rendered more digestible in the stomach by the addition of vinegar, although it is difficult to offer either a chemical or physiological explanation of the fact. The native vege-

table acids may also be occasionally substituted: the addition of lemon juice to rich and glutinous soups, renders them less liable to disagree with the stomach ; and the custom of eating apple-sauce with pork is, undoubtedly, indebted for its origin to the same cause.

141. THE AROMATIC CONDIMENTS comprise the foreign spices, as pepper, cayenne pepper, cinnamon, nutmeg, cloves, ginger; and the indigenous herbs and roots, such as parsley, thyme, sage, garlic, leek, onion, horseradish, mustard, &c. The former of these were not intended by nature for the inhabitants of temperate climes; they are heating, and highly stimulant.* I am, however, not anxious to give more weight to this objection than it deserves. Man is no longer the child of nature, nor the passive inhabitant of any particular region : he ranges over every part of the globe, and elicits nourishment from the productions of every climate. It may be therefore necessary that he should accompany the ingestion of foreign aliment with foreign condiment.† If we go to the East for tea, there is no reason why we should not go to the West for sugar. The dyspeptic invalid, however, should be cautious in their use ; they may afford temporary benefit at the expense of permanent mischief. It has been well said, that the best quality of spices is to stimulate the appetite, and their worst to destroy, by insensible degrees, the tone of the stomach. The intrinsic goodness of meats should always be suspected, when they require spicy seasoning to compensate for their natural want of sapidity.

---

* Nature is very kind in favouring the growth of those productions which are most likely to answer our local wants. Those situations, for instance, which engender endemic diseases, are in general congenial to the growth of the plants that operate as antidotes to them.—*Pharmacologia*, vol. i. p. 148.

† Swift observes, that such is the extent of modern epicurism, that " *the world must be encompassed before a washerwoman can sit down to breakfast.*"

But, mischievous as the abuse of aromatic condiments may
be, it is innocent in comparison with the custom of swallowing a quantity of brandy to prevent the upbraiding of
our stomachs, or an increased libation of wine to counteract the distress which supervenes a too-copious meal—as
if drunkenness were an antidote to gluttony.

142. OIL. This, with butter, constitutes what is called
the oleaginous condiments. Melted butter is, perhaps,
the most injurious of all the inventions of cookery : oil,
when used in extremely small quantities, as a seasoning to
salads, appears to prevent their running into fermentation,
and consequently obviates flatulency.

OF DRINKS.

143. As the introduction of solid aliment into the stomach is for the purpose of furnishing materials for the
repair of the different textures of the body, so is a supply
of liquid matter essentially necessary to replace those
various fluids which are constantly ejected from the body,
during the exercise of its different functions. The necessity of this supply, as well as its quantity, are both indicated by a certain feeling which the want of it excites,
named *thirst*. In this point of view, therefore, the drinks
ought to be considered as real aliments; and, indeed, it
is a question whether they may not also undergo certain
decompositions in the body, and be made to surrender
elements for the formation of solid parts.* The chyme
and chyle may also require the assistance of some liquid
medium to favour the absorption of its finer and more
nutritive parts, which, by increasing the fluidity of the
mass, will expedite the numerous combinations it is
destined to undergo. In every point of view, therefore,

---

* Fish, especially the cetaceous tribe, decompose water, and live
upon its hydrogen.

dilution is an essential operation; and an animal will not only endure the sensation of hunger with more tranquillity than that of thirst, but he will survive longer under the privation of solid than of liquid aliment.* Unfortunately, however, those instincts which nature implanted in us for our guidance have been eradicated by the habits of artificial life: thirst is so rarely experienced, that the very sensation is associated with the idea of disease. The consequence is, that we have been abandoned to the control of our caprice in the selection and use of these agents,— a circumstance which has given origin to numerous disorders. The quantity of diluents which each person may require, will depend upon individual peculiarity, climate, nature of the solid aliment, &c.

144. In appreciating the effects of liquids upon the human body, there are several circumstances independent of the quality of the fluid which deserve some notice; such as temperature, volume, and the period of potation. Although fluids of the usual temperature of the air are grateful and congenial to a healthy stomach, persons disposed to dyspepsia frequently require them to be raised to the temperature of the body; for the stomach, not having sufficient vital energy to establish the re-action which the sudden impression of cold produces in a healthy condition, falls into a state of collapse, and is consequently unable to proceed in the performance of its requisite duties.† It

---

* REDI (*Osservaz. intorno agli Anim. viventi, &c. No.* 34) instituted a series of experiments, with the sole view of ascertaining how long animals can live without food. Of a number of capons which he kept without either solid or liquid aliment, not one survived the ninth day; but one to which he allowed water drank it with avidity, and did not perish until the twentieth day. See our work on MEDICAL JURISPRUDENCE, Art. "*Death by Starvation,*" vol. ii. p. 67.

† This remark applies particularly to the residents of hot climates, whose stomachs are always more or less enfeebled. It appears that the Romans were in the habit of drinking tepid potations at their meals. See Juvenal, Sat. V. v. 63.

deserves notice, however, that fluids heated much above the temperature of the body are equally injurious : it is true that they will frequently, from their stimulus, afford present relief ; but it will always be at the expense of future suffering, and be compensated by subsequent debility. Iced fluids should not be taken, under any circumstances, by those who have delicate stomachs, especially after a meal, the digestion of which is thus retarded, or wholly prevented.

145. It is a popular idea that hot liquids injure the teeth. I entertain great doubts upon the subject. Ribe, in a paper published in the *Amœnitates Academicæ,* observes, that " Man is the only animal accustomed to hot food, and almost the only one affected with carious teeth." This is far from being true ; the term of life in all the graminivorous classes appears to be principally limited by the decay of the teeth, and forms an insuperable obstacle to the prolongation of their existence much beyond the term when they have attained to the perfection of their kind.*

146. The quantity or volume of liquid taken at once into the stomach is a circumstance of material consequence. The reader must refer to that part of the work in which the digestion of drinks is explained (81), in order to understand the importance of the considerations which this question embraces. It is evident that, if the stomach be distended with fluid, the digestion of its solid contents must meet with considerable impediment ; while, at the same time, it is said that the gastric juice becomes too

* In the elephant, who rivals, or perhaps exceeds, man in duration of life, a peculiar provision is found to exist for the purpose of renewing the teeth. The grinding teeth, or *molares,* of the elephant, which consist each of a single piece of bone, intermingled with enamel, are so constructed as to continue growing from behind, in proportion as they are worn away in front by the process of mastication ; so that their duration is coeval with that of the animal.

dilute to fulfil the objects of its secretion. Upon this point I entertain some doubt; the secretions of the stomach are not very soluble in water; and it has been already stated (25) with what extreme difficulty the coagulating quality of the gastric membrane is removed by washing. Be this, however, as it may, it is evident, that if the solid matter be diffused through a large quantity of liquid, it cannot be acted upon by the gastric juice; nor can it be converted into that pultaceous mass which appears to be a preliminary step to its digestion. On the other hand, if the food be too hard or dry, its necessary change by the *churning* of the stomach cannot be accomplished, and the progress of digestion will be impeded. It therefore follows, that different aliments will require different quantities of liquid to assist their chymification. Animal food demands, of course, a greater quantity of drink than vegetable food; roasted than boiled meat; and baked still more than roasted.—The next question to be considered is, as to the most suitable period for taking liquids: and this is, in some measure, answered by the preceding observations. By drinking *before* a meal, we place the stomach in a very unfit condition for the duties it has to perform. By drinking *during* a meal, we shall assist digestion, if the solid matter be of a nature to require it; and impede it, if the quantity taken renders the mass too liquid. Those physicians, therefore, who have insisted upon the necessity of a total abstinence of liquid during a meal, appear to have forgotten that every general rule must be regulated by circumstances. The best test of its necessity is afforded by the sensations of the individual, which ought not to be disregarded merely because they appear in opposition to some preconceived theory. The valetudinarian who, without the feeling of thirst, drinks during a meal because he has heard that it assists digestion; and he who abstains from liquid, in opposition to this feeling, in consequence of the clamour which

the partisans of a popular lecturer have raised against the
custom; will equally err, and contribute to the increase of
the evil they so anxiously seek to obviate.   Dr. W. Philip
has stated a fact, the truth of which my own experience
justifies, that " eating too fast causes thirst; for the food
being swallowed without a due admixture of saliva, the
mass formed in the stomach is too dry." I may conclude
these remarks by observing, that as hunger and thirst are,
to a certain extent, incompatible sensations, it is probable
that nature intended that the appetite for food should first
be satisfied, before a supply of drink becomes necessary;
and if our food possess that degree of succulence which
characterises digestible aliment, there will be no occasion
for it.   But, under any circumstances, the quantity taken
should be small: it is during the intervals of our solid
meals that the liquid necessary for the repair of our fluids
should be taken; and both theory and experience appear
in this respect to conform, and to demonstrate the advantage which attends a liquid repast about four or five hours
after the solid meal.   At about this period the chyle has
entered its proper vessels, and is flowing into the blood, in
order to undergo its final changes.   Then it is that the
stomach, having disposed of its charge, receives the wholesome draught with the greatest advantage; then it is that
the blood, impregnated with new materials, requires the
assistance of a diluent to complete their sanguification,
and to carry off the superfluous matter; and it is then that
the kidneys and the skin will require the aid of additional
water to assist the performance of their functions.   The
common beverage of tea, or some analogous repast, originally suggested no doubt by an instinctive desire for liquid
at this period, is thus sanctioned by theory, while its advantages are established by experience.

147. WATER is unquestionably the natural beverage of
man; but any objection against the use of other beverages,
founded on their artificial origin, I should at once repel by

the same argument (4) which has been adduced in defence
of cookery.   We are to consider man as he is, not as he
might have been, had he never forsaken the rude path of
nature.   I am willing to confess, that " the more simply
life is supported, and the less stimulus we use, the better ;
and that he is happy who considers water the best drink,
and salt the best sauce :" but how rarely does a physician
find a patient who has regulated his life by such a maxim!
He is generally called upon to reform stomachs, already
vitiated by bad habits, and which cannot, without much
discipline, be reconciled to simple and healthy aliment.
Under such circumstances, nothing can be more injudicious
than abruptly to withdraw the accustomed stimuli, unless
it can be shewn that they are absolutely injurious ; a question which it will be my duty to investigate hereafter.

148. The qualities of water differ essentially, according
to the source from which it has been obtained ; and those
accustomed to this beverage are sensible to differences
which wholly escape the observation of less experienced
judges.   How far the existence of foreign matter injures
its salubrity, has been a subject of much controversy : the
truth, perhaps, lies between the extremes ; those who insist
upon the necessity of distillation for its purification, and
those who consider every description of water as alike
salubrious, are, in my opinion, equally remote from truth.
That the presence of minute quantities of earthy matter
can become a source of disease, appears absurd ; while it
would be highly dangerous to deny the morbid tendency
of water that holds putrescent animal or vegetable matter
in solution, or which abounds in mineral impregnation.

149. The usual varieties of common water were classed
and defined by Celsus, and modern chemists have not
found any reason to reject the arrangement—" *Aqua le-
vissima pluvialis est; dein fontana, tum ex flumine, tum ex
puteo; posthæc ex nive aut glacie, gravior his ex lacu; gra-
vissima ex palude.*"

1. RAIN WATER, when collected in the open fields, is certainly the purest natural water, being produced as it were by a natural distillation. When, however, it is collected near large towns, it derives some impregnation from the smoky and contaminated atmosphere through which it falls; and, if allowed to come in contact with the houses, will be found to contain calcareous matter; in which case it ought never to be used without being previously boiled and strained. Hippocrates gave this advice; and M. Margraaf, of Berlin, has shewn the wisdom of the precaution by a satisfactory series of experiments.

2. SPRING WATER, in addition to the substances detected in rain water, generally contains a small portion of muriate of soda, and frequently other salts: but the larger springs are purer than the smaller ones; and those which occur in primitive countries, and in siliceous rocks, or beds of gravel, necessarily contain the least impregnation. An important practical distinction has been founded upon the fact, that the water of some springs dissolves soap, while that of others decomposes and curdles it: the former has been termed *soft*, the latter *hard*, water. Soft water is a more powerful solvent of all vegetable matters, and is consequently to be preferred for domestic as well as medicinal purposes. The brewer knows well from experience, how much more readily and copiously *soft* water will dissolve the extractive matter of his malt; and the housewife does not require to be told, that *hard* water is incapable of making good tea. Sulphate of lime is the salt which generally imparts the quality of hardness to water; and it has been said that its presence will sometimes occasion an uneasy sense of weight in a weak stomach. The quantity

of this salt varies considerably; but, in general, it appears that the proportion of five grains in a pint of water will constitute *hardness,* unfit for washing with soap, and for many other purposes of domestic use. Animals appear to be more sensible of the impurities of water than man. Horses, by an instinctive sagacity, always prefer soft water; and when, by necessity or inattention, they are confined to the use of that which is *hard,* their coats become rough and ill-conditioned, and they are frequently attacked with the gripes. Pigeons are also known to refuse hard, after they have been accustomed to soft water.*

3. RIVER WATER. This, being derived from the conflux of numerous springs with rain water, generally possesses considerable purity; that the proportion of its saline contents should be small, is easily explained by the precipitation which must necessarily take place from the union of different solutions : it is, however, liable to hold in suspension particles of earthy matter, which impair its transparency, and sometimes its salubrity. This is particularly the case with the Seine, the Ganges, and the Nile :† but as the impurities are, for the most part, only suspended, and not truly dissolved, mere rest or filtration will therefore restore to it its original purity. The chemist, therefore, after such a process, would be unable to distinguish water taken

---

* Hard water has certainly a tendency to produce disease in the spleen of certain animals, especially in sheep. This is the case on the eastern side of the island of Minorca, as we are informed by Cleghorn.

† Alpini informs us, that elephantiasis is endemial in Egypt, which Galen ascribes to the impure water of the Nile; an opinion which is adopted by Lucretius :

> " Est elephas morbus, qui propter flumina Nili
> Gignitur Ægypto in medio."

up at London from that procured at Hampton-
court. There exists a popular belief, that the
water of the Thames is peculiarly adapted for the
brewery of porter; it is only necessary to observe,
that such water *is never* used in the London brew-
eries. The vapid taste of river, when compared
with spring water, depends upon, the loss of air and
carbonic acid, from its long exposure.

4. WELL WATER is essentially the same as spring
water, being derived from the same source; it is,
however, more liable to impurity from its stagnation
or slow infiltration :* hence our old wells furnish
much purer water than those which are more recent,
as the soluble particles are gradually washed away.
Mr. Dalton observes, that the more any spring is
drawn from, the softer the water will become.

5. SNOW WATER has been supposed to be unwholesome, and in particular to produce bronchocele, from
the prevalence of that disease in the Alps: but it
does not appear upon what principle its insalubrity
can depend. The same strumous affection occurs
at Sumatra, where ice and snow are never seen;
while, on the contrary, the disease is quite unknown
in Chili and Thibet, although the rivers of those
countries are supplied by the melting of the snow
with which the mountains are covered. The same
observations will apply to *ice water.* The trials of
Captain Cook, in his voyage round the world, prove
its wholesomeness beyond a doubt: in the high
southern latitudes he found a salutary supply of
fresh water in the ice of the sea. " This melted
ice," says Sir John Pringle, " was not only sweet
but soft, and so wholesome as to shew the fallacy

---

* Dr. Percival observes, that bricks harden the softest water, and
give it an aluminous impregnation: the common practice of lining wells
with them is therefore very improper, unless they be covered with cement.

of human reasoning, unsupported by experiments."
When immediately melted, snow water contains no
air, as it is expelled during the act of freezing, consequently it is remarkably vapid; but it soon re-
covers the air it had lost, by exposure to the atmosphere.

6. LAKE WATER is a collection of rain, spring, and
river waters, contaminated with various animal
and vegetable matter, which from its stagnant nature have undergone putrefaction in it. This objection may be urged with greater force against the
use of water collected in ponds and ditches, and
which the inhabitants of some districts are often
under the necessity of drinking. I have known
an endemic diarrhœa to arise from such a circumstance.

7. MARSH WATER, being the most stagnant, is the
most impure of all water, and is generally loaded
with decomposing vegetable matter. There can
be no doubt, that numerous diseases have sprung
up from its use.

150. It is, however, in vain that pure water is discovered, if proper means be not adopted to convey it for the
use of the inhabitants. In ancient times this was done
by means of aqueducts of extraordinary magnificence; and
the materials of which they were composed were even
then acknowledged to be capable of affecting the water
which flowed through them. Palladius testifies his aversion to the use of lead, as apt to become covered with
cerusse, and thereby rendered poisonous; and Vitruvius
and Columella recommend pipes of earthenware, as not
only cheaper but *more wholesome* than those of lead. Dr.
Lambe, to whom we are indebted for an important work*

---

* Researches into the Properties of Spring Water, with Medical
Cautions against the Use of Lead.

upon this subject, states, that there is a great diversity in the corrosive powers of different waters : in some places the use of leaden pumps has been discontinued, from the expense entailed upon the proprietors by the perpetual want of repair.   Dr. Lambe states an instance where the proprietor of a well ordered his plumber to make the lead of a pump of double the thickness of the metal usually employed on such occasions, to save the charge of repairs; because he had observed that *the water was so hard,* as he called it, *that it corroded the lead very soon.* If any acidity be communicated to the water, from the accidental intrusion of decayed leaves or other vegetable matter, its power of dissolving this metal will be increased to a very dangerous extent.   The noted colic of Amsterdam is said by Tronchin, who has written a history of the epidemic, to have been occasioned by leaves falling and putrefying in leaden cisterns filled with rain water.   Van Swieten has also related an instance of a whole family who were afflicted with colic from a similar cause ; * and Dr. Lambe entertains no doubt, but that the very striking case recorded in the Medical Commentaries† proceeded more from some foulness in the cistern, than from the solvent power of the water.   In this instance, the officers of a packet vessel used water out of a leaden cistern; the men also drank the same water, except that the latter had been kept in wood : the consequence was, that all the officers were seized with colic, while the men remained healthy.   Sir George Baker has furnished the following striking illustration of this subject :—" The most remarkable case that now occurs to my memory," says he, " is that of Lord Ashburnham's family, in Sussex; to which spring water was supplied from a considerable distance in leaden pipes. In consequence, his lordship's servants were every year tormented with colic, and some of them died. An eminent

* Van Swieten ad Boerhaav. Aphor. 1060, Comment.
† Duncan Med. Comment., Dec. 2, 1794.

physician of Battle, who corresponded with me on the subject, sent up some gallons of that water, which were analysed by Dr. Higgins, who reported that the water had contained more than the common proportion of carbonic acid; and that he found in it lead in solution, which he attributed to the action of the carbonic acid. In consequence of this representation, Lord Ashburnham substituted wooden for leaden pipes; and from that time his family have experienced no particular complaints in their bowels." As timber pipes are liable to decay, and to impart a bad taste to the water, those made of cast-iron are to be greatly preferred.

151. For the purification and preservation of water, numerous methods have been adopted. The mechanical impurities may be removed by filtration, a process which is suggested by nature herself; for all springs arising through sand, gravel, &c., must undergo this process. Hence it occurred, that if waters of a putrid, marshy, or unwholesome nature, were filtered through a factitious bed of sand, or a vessel made of porous stone,* they might be deprived of their bad qualities. As that peculiar property of water which constitutes what is termed *hardness* generally depends upon the presence of *sulphate of lime* in solution, it cannot be removed by simple filtration; but the addition of an alkaline carbonate† twenty-four hours before it is used, will be found to restore it; or, if it should depend upon *super-carbonate of lime*, long ebullition, without any addition, will be found sufficient for its cure. Another mode of improving water, and the one that has been most recently discovered, is by means of charcoal, a substance which enjoys, in an eminent degree, the property of preserving water from corruption, and of purifying it

---

* Various machines have been constructed for this purpose; but the most modern, and, in my opinion, the best, is that known by the name of " Bennet's Patent Filtering Machine."

† In the proportion of from ten to fifteen grains to every pint.

after it has been corrupted : hence the filtration of water through alternate layers of sand and charcoal offers a ready and effectual mode of abstracting its impurities, especially when they consist of animal or vegetable matter. Where we have reason, however, to suspect much injurious contamination, the process of boiling should never be omitted; after which it may be strained and filtered, and lastly agitated in contact with the atmosphere, in order to restore to it its natural proportion of air. In China, water is never drank until it has been boiled. The mischievous effects of impure water, where it cannot be corrected by any chemical process, are said to be best counteracted by some bitter vegetable. Virey supposes that this circumstance first induced the Chinese to infuse the leaves of the tea plant.

152. The juices and infusions of vegetable and animal matter constitute the second division of drinks.

153. TOAST WATER. By impregnating water with the soluble parts of toasted bread, it will frequently agree with those stomachs which rebel against the use of the pure fluid. It is thus rendered slightly nutritive, holding a certain portion of gum and starch in solution. Sir A. Carlisle recommends that it should be prepared with hard biscuit, reduced by fire to a coffee colour. This drink, he says, being free from yeast, is a most agreeable beverage. Much depends upon the water being at a boiling temperature, and it ought to be drank as soon as it has cooled sufficiently ; for, by keeping, it acquires an unpleasant flavour. Infusions of other kinds of bread, in particular of toasted oat-cakes, also dried or toasted oatmeal, have been recommended ; but the taste of such infusions would not be palatable to any one who has not been accustomed to oat-bread.

154. BARLEY WATER. The decoction of barley is a very ancient beverage ; it is recommended by Hippocrates, and preferred by him to every other aliment in acute

diseases. Barley has the advantage over other grains, in affording less viscid potations. The invention of *pearl barley* has greatly increased the value of this grain; it is prepared by the removal of its husk or cuticle, and afterwards by being rounded and polished in a mill. These well-known granules consist chiefly of fecula, with portions of mucilage, gluten, and sugar, which water extracts by decoction; but the solution soon passes into the acetous fermentation. The bran of barley contains an acrid resin, and it is to get rid of such an ingredient that it is deprived of its cuticle. The addition of lemon juice and sugar-candy greatly improve the flavour of this drink.

155. GRUEL. Oats, when freed from their cuticle, are called *groats;* in which state, as well as when ground into meal, they yield to water, by coction, the fecula they contain, and form a nutritious gruel, which has also the property of being slightly aperient. It should never be kept longer than forty-eight hours, as it becomes acescent after that period. Gruel may be made of a different degree of consistence, according to the object of its potation. If it be used as a demulcent drink, it should be thin; and may be made, as Dr. Kitchener, our culinary censor, informs us, by mixing well together, by degrees, in a pint basin, *one* table-spoonful of oatmeal with three of cold water, and then adding carefully a pint of boiling water, which is to be boiled for five minutes, stirring it all the time, to prevent the oatmeal from burning at the bottom of the stewpan; then strain through a hair sieve, to separate the undissolved parts of the meal from the gruel. If a more substantial repast is required, double the above quantity of oatmeal must be treated in a similar manner. To increase the nutritive quality of this aliment, broth or milk may be substituted for water. Some persons are in the habit of introducing a piece of butter into gruel; but the propriety of this practice is questionable, where the stomach is disposed to generate acidity.

156. SAGE TEA. The virtues of sage have been so extravagantly praised, that, like many of our remedies,* the plant has fallen into disuse from the disgust which its panegyrists have excited. I am convinced, however, that in the form of infusion it possesses some power in allaying the irritability of the stomach,† and that, on many occasions, it will furnish a salutary beverage. The same observation will apply to *balm tea.*

157. TEA. There is no subject which has occasioned a greater controversy amongst dietetic writers than the subject of tea. By one party it is decried as a poison; by another it is extolled as a medicine, and a valuable addition to our food ; while some refer all its beneficial effects to the water thus introduced into the system, and its evil consequences to the high temperature at which it is drank. In order to understand the value of the different arguments which have been adduced in support, or to the disparagement, of this beverage, it will be necessary to inquire into its composition. Two kinds of tea are imported into this country, distinguished by the epithets *black* and *green.* Both contain astringent and narcotic principles, but in very different proportions; the latter producing by far the most powerful influence upon the nervous system. As the primary operation of every narcotic is stimulant, tea is found to exhilarate and refresh us, although there exist individuals who are so morbidly sensible to the action of certain bodies of this class, that feelings of depression, accompanied with various nervous sensations and an unnatural vigilance, follow the potation of a single cup of strong tea; while others experience, from the same cause, symptoms indicative of derangement of the digestive organs: but these are exceptions from which no general rule ought to be deduced. The salubrity of the infusion to

* Pharmacologia, vol. i. p. 35.

† It is frequently used by the Chinese as a tonic for debility of the stomach.

the general mass of the community is established by sufficient testimony to outweigh any argument founded on
individual cases. It must, however, be admitted, that
if this beverage be taken too soon after dinner, the
digestion of the meal may be disturbed by the distension
it will occasion, as well as by its influence as a diluent;
the narcotic and astringent principles may also operate in
arresting chymification : but when a physician gives it his
sanction, it is with the understanding that it shall be
taken in moderate quantities, and at appointed seasons.
When drank four hours after the principal meal, it will
assist the ulterior stages of digestion, as already explained
(146), and promote the insensible perspiration; while it
will afford to the stomach a grateful stimulus after its
labours. With regard to the objection urged against its
use, on the ground of temperature, it will be only necessary to refer to the observations which have been already
offered upon this subject (144). In enumerating, however,
the advantages of tea, it must not be forgotten that it has
introduced and cherished a spirit of sobriety; and it must
have been remarked by every physician of general practice,
that those persons who dislike tea, frequently supply its
place by spirit and water. The addition of milk certainly
diminishes the astringency of tea; that of sugar may
please the palate, but cannot modify the virtues of the
infusion.

158. COFFEE. The hostility which has been mani-
fested against the use of tea, has been extended, with
equal rancour, against that of coffee; and, probably, with
equal injustice. The principle upon which its qualities
depend is more stimulant than that of tea, and certainly
exerts a different species of action upon the nervous system,
although it is very difficult to define the nature of this
difference. If taken immediately after a meal, it is not
found to create that disturbance in its digestion which
has been noticed as the occasional consequence of tea; on

the contrary, it accelerates the operations of the stomach, and will frequently enable the dyspeptic to digest sub- stances, such as fat and oily aliment, which would other- wise occasion much disturbance. The custom of taking coffee immediately after dinner, as so universally practised by the French, no doubt must counteract the evil effects which the peculiar form of their diet is calculated to pro- duce. Coffee, like tea, has certainly an antisoporific effect on many individuals; it imparts an activity to the mind which is incompatible with sleep: but this will rarely occur if the beverage be taken for several hours before our accustomed period of repose. It seems to be generally admitted, that it possesses the power of counteracting the effects of narcotics; and hence it is used by the Turks with much advantage, in abating the influence of the inordinate quantities of opium they are accustomed to swallow. Where our object is to administer it as a pro- moter of digestion, it should be carefully made by infusion; decoction dissipates its aroma. The addition of milk is one of questionable propriety; that of sugar, or rather sugar- candy, may be allowed.* I have known some persons who have never taken this beverage without suffering from acidity in the stomach : where this happens, the practice must be abandoned.

159. CHOCOLATE. In consequence of the large quan- tity of nutritive matter which this liquid contains, it should

---

* Coffee has been often imitated by the torrefaction of various grains. In the " *Fourth Century of Observations*," in the " *Miscellanea Curiosa*," we find a critical dissertation on the coffee of the Arabians, and on Euro- pean coffee, or such as may be prepared from grain or pulse. Dillenius gives an account of his own preparations made with peas, beans, and kidney-beans ; but says that made of rye comes nearest to true coffee, and was with difficulty distinguished from it. This fact is curious, inas- much as a spurious coffee has been lately vended, which is nothing more than roasted rye. The article is well known, under the name of " HUNT's ECONOMICAL BREAKFAST POWDER."

be regarded rather as food than drink. It is prepared by reducing the cocoa nut into paste, with sugar, milk, or eggs: it is also frequently mixed with different aromatics, the most common of which is the *vanilla,* a substance very liable to disagree with the stomach, and to produce a train of nervous symptoms. As a common beverage, chocolate is highly objectionable; it contains an oil which is difficult of assimilation; it therefore oppresses the stomach: this effect is of course increased by the application of too much heat in its preparation. Another objection against its use is to be found in the observations which I have already offered upon the subject of too great concentration (117).

160. Cocoa is usually considered as a substitute for chocolate. As it contains less nutritive matter, it is not so objectionable; and, as the oily matter exists only in small quantities, it is less likely to disagree with the stomach.

161. Whey is a delightful beverage; but as its nature and operation cannot be well understood until the composition of milk is investigated, the observations which I have to offer upon its use will be deferred until the history of that fluid has been examined.

162. The nature of weak broths, and the manner in which they are decomposed in the digestive organs, have been already considered (83); and I shall have occasion to revert to the subject in a future part of the work.

163. There are certain saline solutions which are frequently employed as drinks, and deserve some attention in this place : such are *imperial* and *soda water.*

164. Imperial. This is a solution of cream of tartar flavoured with lemon peel. It ought never to be used except as a medicine. If employed as an ordinary drink, it is apt to retard digestion. If ever useful as an article of diet, it will be under circumstances of robust health, and where a large quantity of animal food has been taken.

165. Soda Water. The modern custom of drinking this inviting beverage during, or immediately after dinner,

has been a pregnant source of dyspepsia. By inflating the stomach at such a period, we inevitably counteract those muscular contractions of its coats which are essential to chymification. The quantity of soda thus introduced scarcely deserves notice: with the exception of the *carbonic acid gas,** it may be regarded as water, more mischievous only in consequence of the exhilarating quality inducing us to take it at a period at which we should not require the more simple fluid.

FERMENTED LIQUORS.

166. Volumes have been written to prove that spirit, in every form, is not only unnecessary to those who are in health, but that it has been the prolific source of the most painful and fatal diseases to which man is subject; in short, that Epimetheus himself did not, by opening the box of Pandora, commit a greater act of hostility against our nature than the discoverer of fermented liquors. Every apartment, it is said, devoted to the circulation of the glass, may be regarded as a temple set apart for the performance of human sacrifices; and that they ought to be fitted up, like the ancient temples of Egypt, in a manner to shew the real atrocity of the superstition that is carried on within their walls. This is mere rant and nonsense; a striking specimen of the fallacy of reasoning against the *use* of a custom from its *abuse*. There exists no evidence to prove that a temperate use of good wine, when taken at seasonable hours, has ever proved injurious to healthy adults. In youth, and still more in infancy,† the stimulus

---

* Late discoveries have shewn, that the carbonic acid exists in a liquid state in soda water; when, therefore, it is hastily swallowed, it robs the stomach of a certain portion of heat, as it passes from a liquid into a gaseous state. It therefore cools as well as distends that organ.

† An ingenious surgeon tried the following experiment.—He gave to two of his children, for a week alternately, after dinner, to the one a full

which it imparts to the stomach is undoubtedly injurious; but there are exceptions even to this general rule. The occasional use of *diluted** wine has improved the health of a child, by imparting vigour to a torpid stomach : we ought, however, to consider it rather as a medicine than as a luxury.

167. Without entering farther into the discussion of a question which has called so many opponents into the field, it may be observed, that whatever opinion we may have formed as to the evils or advantages consequent upon the invention of wine, we are not called upon, as physicians, to defend it; our object is to direct remedies for the cure of those diseases which assail man as we find him in the habits of society, not as he might have been had he continued to derive his nourishment from the roots of the earth, and his drink from its springs. As these habits, says Dr. W. Philip, are such, that more or less alcohol is necessary to support the usual vigour of the greater number of people, even in health, nothing could be more injudicious than wholly to deprive them of it when they are already weakened by disease, unless it could be shewn that even a moderate use of it essentially adds to their disease, which, in dyspeptics, is by no means the case. My own experience coincides with that of Dr. W. Philip. In cases where the vinous stimulant has been withdrawn, I have generally witnessed an aggravation of the dyspeptic symptoms, accompanied with severe depression of spirit :

glass of Sherry, and to the other a large China orange. The effects that followed were sufficient to prove the injurious tendency of vinous liquor. In the one the pulse was quickened, the heat increased, the urine became high coloured, and *the stools destitute of the usual quantity of bile;* whilst the other had every appearance that indicated high health. The same effects followed when the experiment was reversed. See *Beddoes's Hygeia,* vol. ii. p. 35.

* By diluting the wine, we apply the stimulus more generally to the stomach, and thus produce a greater effect with a less quantity of spirit.

like Sindbad, in the Arabian tale, the patient has borne a weight on his shoulders which he has in vain attempted to throw off, until the fermented juice of the grape enabled him to triumph over his enemy.

168. Although it is impossible to enter at any length on the subject of wine, upon which so many volumes have been already written, a work on dietetics would be very imperfect, were the distinctions which exist between the different species to be left unnoticed. Many of these distinctions are important in a medical point of view, as the chemical circumstances, upon which they depend, confer upon the respective wines qualities which are directly connected with their effects on the body.

169. The term Wine is more strictly and especially applied to express the fermented juice of the *grape;* although, in common language, it is used to denote that of *any* sub-acid fruit. The presence of *tartar* is perhaps the circumstance by which the grape is more strongly distinguished from all the other sub-acid fruits that have been applied to the art of wine-making. Its juice, besides, contains, within itself, all the principles essential to vinification, in such a proportion and state of balance as to enable it, at once, to undergo a regular and complete fermentation; whereas, the juices of other fruits require artificial additions for this purpose : and the scientific application, and due adjustment of these means, constitute the art of making domestic wines.* It has been remarked, that all those wines that contain an excess of malic acid are of a bad quality : hence the grand defect that is necessarily inherent in the wines of this country, and which leads them to partake of the properties of cider; for in the

---

* For an account of which, the reader is referred to a most ingenious and interesting essay by Dr. Macculloch, entitled " Remarks on the Art of making Wine; with Suggestions for the Application of its Principles to the Improvement of Domestic Wines."

place of the *tartaric*, the malic acid always predominates in our native fruits.

170. The characteristic ingredient of all wines is *alcohol;* and the quantity of this, and the condition or state of combination in which it exists, are the circumstances that include all the interesting points of inquiry, and explain the relative effects which different wines produce upon the system. I shall therefore proceed to investigate the various species, with reference to such conditions.

171. Wines may be, at once, resolved into two great divisions; into those which are coloured, and commonly called *red* wines, and into those which have a yellow tinge, more or less deep, termed *white* wines. This colouring matter is not derived from the juice, but from the husk of the grapes. If, therefore, the fermentation be not permitted to take place in contact with the husks, a colourless wine is in all cases produced. This colouring matter is highly astringent, and consequently the red wines differ from the white in their effects upon the stomach; and yet it is difficult to explain the well-known extent of this operation, by the presence of so small a proportion of active matter. It must, however, be remembered, that irritable stomachs are frequently impatient of astringent matter. Many persons are incapable of drinking Port wine, in consequence of the heartburn it occasions; while others, on the contrary, appear to derive advantage from the tonic influence of its astringency. This is a circumstance of idiosyncrasy which no theory can explain. A popular writer remarks, " When my stomach is not in good temper, it generally desires to have *red* wine; but when in best health, nothing affronts it more than to put *Port* in it: and one of the first symptoms of its coming into adjustment, is a wish for *white* wine." Every physician must be practically aware of the caprice which the stomach displays in its morbid conditions; but, as a general rule, it may be stated, that *white* deserve a preference over

red wines, because the latter being pressed, and subjected to a stronger fermentation to extract the colouring principle from the husk, are necessarily more loaded with extractive and astringent matter; and as this remains in the stomach after the liquid portion of the wine is absorbed (83), it will be liable to occasion disturbance.

172. The odour, or *bouquet,* and flavour, which distinguish one wine from another, evidently depend upon some volatile and fugacious principle not hitherto investigated by the chemist; this, in sweet and half-fermented wines, is immediately derived from the fruit, as in those from the *Frontignan* and *Muscat* grapes : but in the more perfect wines, as in *Claret, Hermitage, Rivesaltes,* and *Burgundy,* it bears no resemblance to the natural flavour of the fruit, but is altogether the product of the vinous process. The menstruum of this volatile principle is, doubtless, in most instances, the alcohol contained in wines; but its quantity is so minute as to be incapable of separation. In this latter case it frequently appears to produce a very remarkable effect upon the nervous system, and may, possibly, be hereafter discovered to be a new principle of extraordinary powers : such an opinion, at least, is sanctioned by the well-known effects of Burgundy; the excitement produced by this wine being peculiar, and not bearing any relation to the proportion of alcohol contained in it. Some wines are artificially flavoured by the introduction of foreign ingredients, as by almonds in Madeira wines, as well as in those of Xeres and Saint Lucar; and hence their well-known nutty flavour. Among the ancients, and in modern Greece, it is at this day the fashion to give a resinous flavour, by the introduction of turpentine into the casks. These wines were supposed to assist digestion, to restrain morbid discharges, to provoke urine, and to strengthen the bowels : but Dioscorides informs us, that they were known to produce vertigo, pain

in the head, and many evils not incidental to the potations of the same vinous liquor, when free from such admixtures.

173. The quantity of acid contained in wines has been supposed capable of diminishing their salubrity, and in some cases of rendering them imminently noxious. There can be no doubt, that where acetic acid has been generated during a protracted fermentation, it will deteriorate the virtues of wine, and render it obnoxious to the stomach; but where the acid arises from the nature of the fruit, it cannot merit the odium which popular opinion would assign to it. What, for instance, is the acid contained in Madeira, and against which so many objections have been urged? an atom merely of tartar. And yet the person who fancies that his digestion can be deranged by its action, will swallow twenty times the quantity of the same ingredient in some other shape, with perfect indifference and impunity. Sir Anthony Carlisle,* who has carried his prejudices against acids farther than any other writer, says, " long-continued and watchful observation induce me to conclude, that the acid qualities of fermented liquors are no less injurious than the spirit which they contain." If the process of reasoning, by which he arrived at such a conclusion, be not more correct than the experiments which enabled him to ascertain the quantities of acid matter in different fermented liquors, it cannot merit the confidence of the public. His table, which was constructed to exhibit " gross proofs" (*of error?*) of the relative quantities of free acid in ordinary fermented drinks, is a chemical curiosity. The tyro who has attended a single course of lectures will at once perceive, by casting his eyes over this table, that its results are wholly inconsistent with the doctrine of chemical equivalents. He tells us, that " a moderate-sized glassful, containing two

* An Essay on the Disorders of Old Age.

ounces (avoirdupois) of Port wine, required for neutralization, three grains of Henry's calcined magnesia, or six grains of carbonate of potass, or four grains of sub-carbonate of soda, or nine grains of prepared chalk." Now these are not the relative proportions in which such bases could, by any possibility, unite with any acid ; but, granting, for the sake of argument, that our scales of equivalents are in error, and that the true proportions have been ascertained by the experiments in question, we shall then discover, that the tabulated results are not consistent with themselves ; for in a second experiment, made with vidonia, the numbers indicating the combining weights of these substances are not, as in the former case, in the relation of 3, 6, and 4, but in that of 5; 7; and 6 ; in the third experiment with Sherry, in that of 3, 5, and 4; in a fourth with London porter, in that of 5, 3·5, and 3; and, in the last, with brewers' fresh table beer, the proportions are 2·5, 2, and 2. Sir Anthony was aware of these discordances ; and he attempts to explain them by supposing that they may be "owing to the varying affinities of native acids, derived from the fruits, and the acid products of fermentation, as they regarded the several tests." It is almost unnecessary to state, that this supposition is in direct variance with the acknowledged doctrine of definite proportionals, and the fundamental principle of chemical combinations. Let the acids be what they may, the respective bases must always unite with them in an invariable and constant ratio.

174. Before we quit the subject of vinous acidity, I shall beg to say a few words upon its supposed influence in exciting paroxysms of gout. That such attacks have followed particular potations, I do not mean to deny ; but a slight excess of any kind, whether in diet or in exercise, will excite the disease in those predisposed to it. Where the train is laid, an additional glass of claret may have acted as the match ; but in all such cases, the explosion

would have equally taken place, had, instead of claret, some other exciting cause fired it.

175. The characteristic ingredient of all wines is ALCOHOL; and the quantity of this, and the condition or state of combination in which it exists, are the circumstances in which the medical inquirer is principally interested. The late experiments of Mr. Brande have thrown considerable light upon this subject; although, as in most instances of discovery, they have raised up new doubts and difficulties. Daily experience convinces us, that the same quantity of alcohol applied to the stomach under the form of wine, and in a state of mixture with water, will produce very different effects upon the body, and to an extent which it is difficult to understand. It has, for instance, been demonstrated beyond the reach of doubt, that Port, Madeira, and Sherry contain from one-fourth to one-fifth their bulk of alcohol; so that a person who takes a bottle of either of them, will thus take nearly half a pint of alcohol, or almost a pint of pure brandy! and, moreover, that different wines, although containing the same absolute proportion of spirit, will be found to vary very considerably in their intoxicating powers. No wonder, then, that such results should have staggered the philosopher, who is naturally unwilling to accept any tests of difference from the nervous system, which elude the ordinary resources of analytical chemistry. The conclusion was therefore drawn, that alcohol must necessarily exist in wine in a far different condition from that in which we know it in a separate state; or, in other words, that its elements only could exist in the vinous liquor, and that their union was determined, and, consequently, alcohol produced, by the act of distillation. That it was the *product*, and not the *educt* of distillation, was an opinion which originated with Rouelle, who asserted that alcohol was not completely formed until the temperature was raised to the point of distillation. More lately, the same doctrine was revived and promul-

gated by Fabbroni, in the Memoirs of the Florentine Aca-
demy. Gay Lusac has, however, silenced the partisans of
this theory, by separating the alcohol by distillation, at
the temperature of 66° Fahrenheit; and, by the aid of a
vacuum, it has since been effected at 56°. And to complete the demonstration, Mr. Brande has shewn that, by
precipitating the colouring matter, and some other elements
of the wine, by the *sub-acetate of lead*, and then saturating
the clear liquor with *sub-carbonate of potass*, the alcohol
may be separated without any elevation of temperature;
and he has accordingly, by this ingenious expedient, been
enabled to construct a table, exhibiting the proportions of
spirit which exist in the several kinds of wine. No doubt,
therefore, can any longer be entertained upon the subject;
and the fact of the difference of effect produced by the
same bulk of alcohol, when presented to the stomach in
different states, is to be explained on the supposition that,
in wine, it is not only more intimately mixed with water,
but that it exists in combination with its extractive matter;
in consequence of which, it is incapable of exerting its
full effects before it becomes altered in its properties, or,
in other words, partially *digested;* and this view of the
subject may be fairly urged in explanation of the fact, that
the intoxicating effects of the same wine are liable to vary,
in degree, in the same individual, from the peculiar state
of his digestive organs at the time of its potation.

176. As the results obtained by Mr. Brande are highly
important in a medical point of view, I shall here subjoin
an extract from his table.

TABLE of the quantity of alcohol (sp. gr. ·825), at 60° Fah., in several kinds of wine and other liquors.

Per cent by measure.		Per cent by measure.	
Port, average of six kinds..	23·48	Hock	8·88
Do. highest	25·83	Palm Wine	4·70
Do. lowest.............	21·40	Vin de Grave	12·80
Madeira, highest	24·42	Frontignac..............	12·79
Do. lowest.............	19·34	Cote Roti	12·32
Sherry, average of four kinds	17·92	Rousillon	17·26
Do. highest	19·83	Cape Madeira	18·11
Do. lowest.............	12·25	Cape Muchat...........	18·25
Claret, aver. of three kinds .	14·43	Constantia	19·75
Calcavalla	18·10	Tent	13·20
Lisbon	18·94	Sheraaz	15·52
Malaga	17·26	Syracuse	15·28
Bucellas...............	18·49	Nice	14·63
Red Madeira............	18·40	Tokay	9·88
Malmsey do............	16·40	Raisin Wine...........	25·77
Marsala................	25·87	Grape Wine	18·11
Ditto ....,........	17·26	Currant Wine	20·55
Red Champagne	11·30	Gooseberry Wine	11 64
White do.	12·80	Elder Wine, Cider & Perry	9·87
Burgundy	11·55	Stout	6·80
Ditto	11·95	Ale	8·88
White Hermitage	17·43	Brandy	53·39
Red do...............	12·32	Rum	53·68
Hock	14·37	Hollands	51·60

177. We have hitherto only considered alcohol as it exists in a combined state in wine; but it is essential to state, that the stronger wines of Spain, Portugal, and Sicily, are rendered marketable in this country by the addition of *brandy*, and must consequently contain more or less *uncombined* spirit; but the proportion of which will not bear a ratio to the quantity added, because, at the period of its admixture, a renewed fermentation is produced by the scientific vintner, which will assimilate and combine a certain portion of the foreign spirit with the wine : this manipulation, in technical language, is called "*fretting in.*"

It is to the quantity of *free*, not to that of *combined* spirit, that the injurious effects of such wines are to be attributed. " It is well known," observes Dr. Macculloch, " that diseases of the liver are the most common and the most formidable of those produced by the use of *ardent* spirits." It is equally certain, that no such disorders follow the intemperate use of *pure* wine, however long indulged in: to the concealed and unwitting consumption of spirit, therefore, as contained in the wines generally drunk in this country, is to be attributed the excessive prevalence of those hepatic affections, which are comparatively little known to our continental neighbours.

178. Much has been said upon the effects of new wine upon the stomach, compared with those produced by that which has been long kept. It will be necessary to consider the changes produced in this liquor by being kept. In the first place, red wine gradually deposits a quantity of cream of tartar, in combination with extractive and colouring matter, forming what is commonly called the crust; so that a considerable portion of that matter which is likely to disagree with the stomach is thus removed: but when kept in the cask, in addition to this change, a quantity of water is evaporated, and the wine becomes comparatively stronger. The custom of exposing Madeira to motion, and a certain elevation of temperature, by sending it a voyage to the East Indies, unquestionably improves the flavour, and produces some internal change in the composition of the wine, which the chemist is unable to explain.

179. In a dietetic point of view, wines may be arranged into four classes; viz. 1. SWEET WINES; 2. SPARKLING or EFFERVESCING; 3. DRY and LIGHT; 4. DRY and STRONG.

1. SWEET WINES contain the greatest proportion of extractive and saccharine matter, and generally the least ardent spirit, though this is often rather disguised than

absent. As in these wines a proportion of sugar has remained unchanged during the process of vinification, they
must be considered as the results of an imperfect fermentation, and are, in fact, mixtures of wine and sugar ; accordingly, whatever arrests the progress of fermentation, must
have a tendency to produce a sweet wine. Thus, boiling
the *must*, or drying the fruit, will, by partially separating
the natural leaven, and dissipating the water, occasion
such a result, as is exemplified by the manufacture of the
wines of Cyprus, the *Vino Cotto* of the Italians, and the
Vinum Coctum of the ancients ; by that of *Frontignac*, the
rich and luscious wines of *Canary*, the celebrated *Tokay*,
Vino Tinto (Tent of Hungary), the Italian *Montefiascone*,
the Persian *Schiras*, the *Malmsey* wines of Candia, Chio,
Lesbos, and Tenedos, and those of the other islands of the
Archipelago. On account of the sugar contained in such
wines, they are liable to become acescent on weak stomachs ; but where this is not the case, they are, in small
quantities, frequently beneficial to invalids.

2. Sparkling or Effervescing Wines. These
are indebted for their characteristic properties to the presence of carbonic acid ; they rapidly intoxicate, in consequence of the alcohol which is suspended in, or, more
probably, in chemical combination with the gas, being
thus applied in a sudden and very divided state to a large
extent of nervous surface : for the same reason, their
effects are generally as transitory as they are sudden.
Independently of the alcohol thus held in solution in the
carbonic acid, it is probable that some active aromatic
matter is volatilised together with it, and which may
account for the peculiar effects produced on some persons
by Champagne.

3. Dry and Light Wines. These are exemplified by
the more esteemed German wines, as *Hock, Rhenish, Mayne,
Moselle, Necker,* and *Elsass;* and those highly-flavoured
wines, *Burgundy, Claret, Hermitage,* &c. The former of

these wines combine the effect of an acid with that of the spirit. They do not contain any uncombined alcohol, and on that account are to be greatly preferred. *Genuine* Claret must be considered as the most beneficial of all our vinous liquors ; it is well fermented ; and, on account of the small proportion of spirit, as well as of extractive, which it contains, it is more salubrious than Port. It has been already observed, that Burgundy appears to hold dissolved some unknown principle of great activity : upon no other supposition can we explain its stimulant properties. A few glasses of this wine will produce heat and headach, which the relative quantity of alcohol in its composition (*see the preceding table*) will not account for.

4. Dry and Strong Wines, as *Madeira, Port, Sherry*, &c. The name *sec*, corruptly written sack, signifies dry. The sec wine, prepared at Xeres, in Spain, is called, accordingly to our orthography, *Sherris*, or *Sherry*. In the manufacture of this wine, *lime** is added to the grapes ; a circumstance, observes Dr. Macculloch, apparently conducive to its well-known dry quality, and which, probably, acts by neutralising a portion of *malic* or *tartaric* acid.

180. It is a fact, not easily explained, that the stomach is frequently outraged by a wine to which it has not been accustomed ; and it is equally true, that a mixture of different wines is a common source of indigestion. The custom of mixing wine with water has its advantages as well as its evils.† By dilution it frequently proves too

---

* The Sack of Shakspeare was probably Sherry; a conjecture which receives additional strength from the following passage :—" You rogue ! here's *lime* in this Sack, too. There is nothing but roguery to be found in villanous man. Yet a coward is worse than a cup of sack with lime in it—a villanous coward !"

† This custom was a favourite practice amongst the ancients. Hence Bacchus was called *Rectus*, because he first introduced it, having taught a certain king of Athens to dilute his wine with water : men, who through

little stimulant to the stomach, and runs into a state of acescency. An invalid is also thus liable to deceive himself, by taking more wine than may be consistent with his welfare. Much, however, depends upon the quality of the wine taken; the lighter wines cannot require dilution, while Port is certainly rendered less injurious by the admixture.

181. Home-made, or domestic wines, may be generally considered as injurious to delicate stomachs; they are apt to ferment, and produce indigestion. Cider and Perry are grateful drinks in hot weather; but as they do not contain a sufficient quantity of spirit to prevent their passing into the acetous fermentation in the stomach of an invalid, they should be avoided by those who have any predisposition to indigestion.

182. BEER. This is an article of beverage in almost every country. The Chinese prepare it from rice, and the Americans from maize. We are also informed by Herodotus, that, in very early history, the art of making a fermented liquor from barley was discovered by the Egyptians. As the climate of England is not congenial to the growth of the vine, this species of liquor is perhaps more universal than in any other country; and it has therefore been denominated *Vinum Britannicum.* In the higher walks of society it has, indeed, of late years, been nearly excluded: but whether this revolution has been attended with advantage, we shall presently have occasion to inquire. Malt liquors differ from wines in several essential

---

drinking staggered before, by mixing water with their wine, began to walk straight. It is also said, in ancient mythology, that the jolly god was educated by the Naiads, or the nymphs of the rivers and fountains; implying, that men ought thence to learn to dilute their wine with water. But a question may arise as to the modification thus produced on the intoxicating powers of wine. I suspect that a quantity of wine, in a state of dilution, will be more intoxicating than an equivalent portion of vinous liquor in a more concentrated form.

points : they contain a much larger proportion of nutritive matter, and a less proportion of spirit; while they contain a peculiar bitter and narcotic principle derived from the hop. It would appear, that the extractive matter furnished by the malt is highly nutritive; and we accordingly find, that those persons addicted to such potations are in general fat.* Where, however, they are indulged in to any extent, without a corresponding degree of exercise, they induce a plethoric state of the body, and all the diseases consequent upon such a condition. In order to understand the process by which they furnish nourishment, I must once more beg to refer the reader to the observations which are offered on the important subject of the digestion of liquids (83); from which it will appear, that a highly-concentrated extract will be left in the stomach after the removal of its watery part. This extract is, for reasons already stated, not very digestible; and will, therefore, require the presence of less inspissated food to promote its chymification. Ale, therefore, when taken without such precautions, is liable to disturb the digestive organs. The addition of the hop increases the value of the liquor, by the grateful stimulus which it imparts, and in some measure redeems it from those vices with which it might otherwise be charged. To those, therefore, whose diet is not very nutritive, ale may be considered not only as an innocent, but as a salubrious article ; and happy is that country, whose labouring classes prefer such a beverage to the mischievous potations of ardent

---

* This fact is so generally admitted by all those who are skilled in the art of TRAINING, that a quantity of ale is taken at every meal by the pugilist who is endeavouring *to screw himself up to his fullest strength.* Jackson, the celebrated trainer, affirms, if any person accustomed to drink wine would but try malt liquor for a month, he would find himself so much the better for it, that he would soon take the one, and abandon the other.

spirit.* These remarks, however, cannot apply to those classes of the community who " fare sumptuously every day." They will not require a nutritive potation of such a character; and light wines have accordingly, in these days of luxury, very properly superseded its use: but I am not disposed to extend this remark to its more humble companion, " *table beer.*" I regard its dismissal from the tables of the great as a matter of regret; its slight, but invigorating bitter, is much better adapted to promote digestion than its more costly substitutes. But it should be soft and mild; for, when stale and hard, it is likely to disturb the bowels, and occasion effects the very opposite to those it is intended to produce. Nor ought it to have too great a proportion of hops, but should be thoroughly fermented and purified. Sydenham always took a glass of small beer at his meals, and he considered it as a preservative against gravel.

183. The great division of malt liquors is into small beer, ale, and porter.

184. The liquor called ALE was originally made of barley, malt, and yeast alone. We are told by one of the oldest English writers on medical subjects (Andrew Boorde†), that those who put in any other ingredient "sophisticated the labour." " It is," he says, " the natural drink of an Englishman; but beer, on the other hand, which is made of malt, hops, and water, is the natural

---

* I certainly do not agree with Dr. Franklin when he states, that the bodily strength furnished by beer can only be in proportion to the solid part of the barley dissolved in the water of which the beer was composed ; and that, as there is a larger proportion of flour in a penny loaf than in a pint of beer, consequently, that more strength is derived from a penny loaf and a pint of water than from a pint of beer. It is the stimulus of the beer that proves so serviceable to the poor man, enabling his stomach to extract more aliment from his innutritive diet.

† The founder of the class of itinerant quacks termed Merry-Andrews; for an account of whom see my Pharmacologia, edit. 6, vol. i. p. 60, *note*.

drink of a Dutchman, and of late is much used in
England, to the great detriment of many Englishmen."
There existed, for a long time, a strong prejudice against
hops, which were considered as " pernicious weeds ;" but
it is now generally admitted, that they constitute the most
valuable ingredient in malt liquors.   Independent of the
flavour and tonic virtues which they communicate, they
precipitate, by means of their astringent principle, the
vegetable mucilage, and thus remove from the beer the
active principle of its fermentation : without hops, therefore, we must either drink our malt liquors new and ropy,
or old and sour.   There are several varieties of ale, distinguishable by their colour : when the malt is slenderly
dried, the ale is *pale ;* or *brown* when the malt is more
roasted, or high-dried.

185. PORTER. This is made from high-dried malt,
and differs from other malt liquors in the proportions of
its ingredients, and from the peculiar manner in which it
is manufactured. Much has been said upon the fraudu-
lent adulteration of this article : but I am inclined to
believe that these statements have been exaggerated. It
is, at all events, certain, that such adulterations are not
carried on in the caldrons of the brewer, but in the barrels
of the publican (see our work on Medical Jurisprudence,
vol. i. p. 375). The origin of the beer called *entire* is to
be thus explained :—Before the year 1730, the malt liquors
in general use in London were ale, beer, and two-penny ;
and it was customary to call for a pint, or tankard, of half-
and-half, *i. e.* half of ale and half of beer, half of ale and
half of two-penny. In course of time, it also became the
practice to call for a pint or tankard of *three-threads,*
meaning a third of ale, beer, and two-penny ; and thus
the publican had the trouble to go to three casks, and
turn three cocks, for a pint of liquor. To avoid this inconvenience and waste, a brewer, of the name of Harwood,
conceived the idea of making a liquor which should par-

take of the same united flavours of ale, beer, and two-penny. He did so, and succeeded, calling it *entire*, or *entire butt*, meaning that it was drawn entirely from one cask or butt; and, as it was a very hearty and nourishing liquor, and supposed to be very suitable for porters and other working people, it obtained the name of " PORTER."

186. ARDENT SPIRITS. The act of extracting alco-holic liquors by distillation from vinous liquors, must be regarded as the greatest curse ever inflicted upon human nature. The fatal effects of dram-drinking have been vividly depicted by numerous writers; and the awful truth has been too frequently illustrated to render any remarks in this place necessary. In a medical point of view, how-ever, spirit may be considered as occasionally useful. Where it is taken in a diluted state, the mixture should always be made twelve hours before it is used. Spirit and water do not easily combine; and much of the force of the former is blunted by intimate incorporation with the latter, as we have already observed, under the history of wine. I throw out this hint to those who are in the habit of drinking weak brandy and water at their meals; although the propriety of such a practice is very questionable. There are cases of dyspepsia, in which wine and beer equally dis-agree with the stomach, producing acidity, and other dis-tressing symptoms : very weak spirit in such a case may, perhaps, be taken with advantage; but its strength should be uniform, and no circumstances should induce the pa-tient to increase the proportion of the spirit. The habit of drinking *liqueurs* cannot be too loudly reprobated : many of these *cordials* are impregnated with narcotic substances, which add to the noxious qualities of the spirit.

An Estimate of the Nutritive and Digestible
Qualities of several Species of Aliment,
as derived from the Application of the
Physiological and Chemical Principles
established in the preceding pages.

Milk, *although fluid, is, in fact, a mixture of solid and
liquid aliment—its chemical composition.— Cream,
Curd, Cheese.— Eggs.— Fish. — Birds. —* Farina-
ceous Aliments; *Bread, &c.— Potatoes.— Rice.—
Pulses.—Fruits.—Of the* Diet of Convalescents.
—Periods for Meals.—*Conduct, to be pursued
previous and subsequent to Meals.— Exercise, Rest,
Sleep.*

187. Were I to follow the steps of all preceding writers
on dietetics, I should present a catalogue of the nutrientia,
and introduce, under each article, a history of its composition and virtues; but the utility of general principles
is to abbreviate labour, and to class under a few heads
those remarks which were previously scattered and unconnected.

188. We have seen that the nutritive qualities of a
substance depend upon its composition; but that its digestibility may be influenced by various mechanical causes
(123). It is by such tests that we have now to examine
the several classes of aliment, and to assign to the individual bodies which they comprehend their relative value
as articles of diet.

189. *Milk.* This is the only nutritive fluid with which
nature has presented us; but if we examine its chemical
composition, we shall soon discover that it possesses
an ingredient which is instantly coagulated in the stomach; so that, in fact, it must be regarded as a mixture of
solid and liquid aliment; the latter, however, considerably

exceeding the former in quantity, and thereby demonstrating the necessity of a greater portion of fluid than of
solid matter, for the reparation of that habitual waste, upon
which the necessity of alimentary supplies is founded.

190. Although recent milk appears as a homogeneous
liquid, it may be resolved, partly by standing, and partly
by agents that do not essentially alter the nature of its
components, into three proximate ingredients, the *cream,
curd,* and *whey.*

   1. The Cream rises to the surface of the milk, after
      it has stood for some hours, and may be skimmed
      off, and thus separated from it. It appears to
      possess many of the properties of oil; is smooth
      and unctuous to the touch, and stains cloth in the
      same manner as other unctuous substances. By
      standing for some days it becomes gradually thicker,
      and at length forms a soft solid, in which the fla-
      vour of cream is no longer perceived, and that of
      cheese is substituted in its place. According to
      the experiments of Berzelius, cream is a compound
      body, consisting of butter, 4·5; cheese, 3·5; and
      whey, 92 parts : but since the whey holds certain
      salts in solution, we may consider the whole of the
      solid matter contained in cream as amounting to
      12·5 per cent. When cream is agitated, as is done
      by the common process of churning, it is separated
      into two parts ; a thick animal oil, well known by
      the name of butter, and a fluid which possesses
      exactly the same properties as milk that has been
      deprived of its cream. This change has been sup-
      posed to be owing to the combination of the cream
      with the oxygen of the atmosphere ; but it takes
      place, though perhaps not equally well, in vessels
      from which the air has been excluded.

   2. Curd. When milk, either deprived or not of its
      cream, is mixed with certain substances, or allowed

to stand until it becomes sour, it undergoes a
change which is called coagulation, consisting in
its separation into a solid substance termed curd,
and a fluid called *whey*. This change may be effected by several agents, such as alcohol, gelatine,
and all astringent vegetables; by acids, and many
neutral salts; by gum, sugar, and more particularly
by the *gastric juice*. The effect is supposed to
arise from the affinity of the coagulating substance
to water, the curd, being principally albumen,
having very little affinity for the same; but this
theory can hardly explain the operation of the
gastric juice: the infusion of a piece of calf's stomach, not larger than a half crown, will coagulate
a quantity of milk sufficient for making a cheese
of sixty pounds weight, although the quantity of
coagulating matter cannot in this case exceed a few
grains.

3. WHEY, or the liquid which remains after the separation of the curd, is a thin and almost transparent
fluid, of a yellowish-green colour, and a pleasant
sweetish taste. It still contains, generally, a portion both of curd and of butter; the former of
which may be separated by a boiling heat, in the
form of coagulum. The buttery matter also sepa-
rates by heat, especially if the whey be previously
allowed to become sour. Whey contains, indeed,
in its recent state, some acetic acid. When whey,
which has been deprived as much as possible from
the butter and curd, is slowly evaporated, it yields
the peculiar substance termed " *sugar of milk*,"
which may be obtained, by clarification with
whites of eggs, in the form of crystals. The presence of this saccharine matter held in solution in
whey enables that fluid to undergo the vinous fermentation; and it is accordingly employed by the

Tartars for making a sort of wine, which is called
Koumiss. For this purpose mare's milk is selected,
as containing a larger proportion of sugar than that
of the cow. Whey also contains several saline
bodies, viz. *muriate of potass, phosphates of lime
and of iron,* and *sulphate of potass;* and a peculiar
animal matter, which gives a precipitate with infusion of galls, and affords carbonate of ammonia
by distillation.

From these investigations, the constituents of
skimmed milk from the cow appear to be as
follow :—

Water.....................	926·75
Curd, with a little cream	28·
Sugar of milk..............	35·
Muriate of potass	1·70
Phosphate of potass	0·25
Lactic acid, acetate of potass with a trace of lactate of iron.................	6·
Earthy phosphates..........	0·30
	1000

191. Although nature has presented us with this compound fluid for the purposes of nourishment, and although
it is evident that its several ingredients are wholesome,
and designed for the various objects of aliment, yet, when
separated by art, they are frequently unwelcome to the
stomach ; that viscus would appear to dislike the interfe-
rence of the cook, in the performance of an analysis which
its own powers are so well calculated to perform. We are
well assured, that the first process which takes place in
the stomach for the chymification of milk, is its separation
into curd and whey ; and yet the former of these substances, when obtained by art, frequently proves highly
oppressive to the stomach, and sometimes occasions ob-

structions in the bowels. CHEESE, again, which is nothing more than the coagulum of milk, pressed, salted,
and partly dried, with a portion of butter, which, having
been enveloped in the curd, is not afterwards separable, is
one of the least digestible of our aliments, and is only
adapted to strong stomachs, and to such persons as use
great and constant exercise. When *toasted,* it is still more
injurious, from acquiring a tenacity of texture highly
hostile to the digestive function of the stomach. BUTTER,
from its oily nature, is apt to disagree with delicate stomachs; and when rendered empyreumatic by heat, produces heartburn, and other distressing symptoms: the use
of hot buttered toast or muffins should, therefore, never
be allowed to dyspeptic invalids. Whey differs considerably in its dietetic value, according to the method employed
for its separation. When this is effected by *rennet,* it
always holds a portion of cream and curd suspended in it,
besides its quantity of sugar. It is, therefore, considerably
nutritive; but it is, at the same time, more acescent than
milk, and hence it is liable to produce flatulence in those
whose stomachs are disposed to encourage fermentation.
Whey that has been produced by spontaneous coagulation
always contains less nutritive matter, is more acid, and
consequently more objectionable, unless, perhaps, as a
drink in certain states of fever.

192. From this account of the composition of milk,
several properties of the entire fluid may be understood.
By boiling it, its albuminous part is not coagulated into a
mass like the white of an egg, on account of the large
quantity of water through which it is diffused; but a thin
pellicle forms on the surface, which, if removed, is immediately replaced by another; and thus the whole of the
albumen may be separated in successive portions. The
effect of this process is therefore to diminish the nutritive
quality of the milk; but it may at the same time render it
more easily digestible. I have known many invalids who

could take boiled milk, who were unable to bear that fluid in its natural state.

193. Milk, in its dietetic relations, may be considered as intermediate between animal and vegetable food; it is easily assimilated, and therefore affords a quick supply of aliment to the system, while it does not excite that degree of vascular action which is produced by other animal matters. Its nutritive powers may be increased by various additions, which have also, on some occasions, the effect of correcting its natural tendency to acidity, and on others, that of obviating the costiveness which it is liable to occasion; such objects are sometimes fulfilled by adding oatmeal gruel to it. In certain states of organic disease, I have found that milk, impregnated with the fatty matter of mutton suet, is a valuable article of diet: such a repast is best prepared by inserting the suet in a muslin bag, and then simmering it with the milk. In common case of dyspepsia it would prove injurious, for the reasons so often alluded to in the course of this work : but where it is an object to introduce much nutritive matter in a small space, I am not acquainted with a better form of aliment. With some practitioners it is a custom to recommend an admixture of lime water with milk, to prevent the acidity which it is apt to create in feeble stomachs. I have occasionally experienced the benefit of such a practice, especially in cases of *tabes mesenterica*.

194. Before quitting this subject, it is necessary to observe, that there exists some difference in the composition of the milk of different animals. That of the human subject is much thinner than cow's milk; is of a bluer colour, and contains much more saccharine matter. It also yields a larger proportion of cream, but from which the butter cannot be separated by agitation. It deposits a part of its curd by mere repose. Asses' milk bears a stronger resemblance to human milk than to any other; it contains

more sugar than that of the cow, and the proportion of curd is so considerable as even to separate on standing, before the milk becomes sour. Goats' milk yields a remarkably thick and unctuous cream, and abounds also in curd.

195. Eggs, in point of nutriment and digestibility, may be classed next to milk; but their qualities will greatly depend upon the manner in which they have been cooked. When raw, they are certainly not so easily digested as when lightly boiled, so as slightly to coagulate their albuminous principle; but if this process be carried too far, they are converted into a hard mass, which requires all the powers of the stomach for its chymification : but this is much accelerated by the use of vinegar as a condiment. They are distinguished by the peculiar quality of singularly affecting some stomachs, even in the smallest quantity; while they do not produce any uneasy impressions on others. I am acquainted with a person who constantly finds an egg to produce uneasiness when his stomach is the least deranged, but who can eat them with impunity at all other times. It is a notorious fact, that eggs, when raw, are laxative, and when cooked are apt to produce costiveness.

FISH.

196. Fish has been generally considered as holding a middle rank between the flesh of warm-blood animals and vegetable food. It is certain that it is less nutritive than mutton or beef; but the health and vigour of the inhabitants of fishing-towns evidently prove that it is sufficiently nourishing for all the purposes of active life : but in order to satisfy the appetite, a large quantity is requisite; and the appetite returns at shorter intervals than those which occur during a diet of meat. Nor does this species of food produce the same stimulus to the body; the pulse is not

strengthened as after a repast of flesh; and that febrile
excitement which attends the digestion of the more nutritive viands is not experienced.   Hence fish affords a most
valuable article of diet to invalids labouring under particular disorders; for it furnishes a chyle moderately nutritive, but, at the same time, not highly stimulant.   From
the nature of its texture, it does not require a laborious
operation of the stomach; although it is sufficiently solid
to rescue it from those objections which have been urged
against liquid or gelatinous food.   From the observations
just offered upon the nutritive powers of fish, it must
follow, that such a diet is not calculated to restore power
to habits debilitated by disease, and should never be directed under such circumstances, but from the conviction
that the digestive powers are unable to convert stronger
aliment into chyle.   The jockeys who *waste themselves* at
Newmarket, in order to reduce their weight, are never
allowed meat, when fish can be obtained.   On account of
the low stimulant power of fish, it requires the assistance
of condiment; and on this account salt appears to be an
essential accompaniment.

197. Fish have been arranged under three divisions;
viz. *fresh-water fish, salt-water fish, and shell fish.*   But,
since the value of these animals as articles of food has an
intimate relation to the colour and texture of their muscles,
and to their gelatinous or oily qualities, it will be expedient
to consider their several varieties, with reference to such
conditions.   Turbot, cod, whiting, haddock, flounder, and
sole, are the least heating of the more nutritive species;
and the flakiness of the fish, and its opaque appearance
after being cooked, may be considered as true indications
of its goodness; for when the muscles remain semi-trans-
parent and bluish, after sufficient boiling, we may reject it
as inferior in value, or not in season.   When the fish is in
high perfection, there is also a layer of white curdy matter,
resembling coagulated albumen, interposed between its

flakes. The whiting is well adapted for weak stomachs, on account of the little viscidity which it possesses ; it is, at the same time, tender, white, and delicate, and conveys sufficient nutriment, with but little stimulus, to the system. The haddock much resembles it, but is firmer in texture. Cod has a more dense fibre than the two former, and contains also more glutinous matter: it is an excellent aliment, but, upon the whole, is not quite so digestible as whiting or haddock. It is generally preferred when large; but such fish are frequently coarse. The haddock is certainly better when it does not exceed a middling size. A process called *crimping* is sometimes adopted, for the purpose of improving cod and some other fish. Sir Anthony Carlisle has investigated the change thus produced; and we are indebted to him for some curious observations upon the subject. Whenever the rigid contractions of death have not taken place, the process may be practised with success. The sea fish, destined for *crimping*, are usually struck on the head when caught, which, it is said, protracts the term of this capability; and the muscles which retain this property longest are those about the head. Many transverse sections of the muscles being made, and the fish immersed in cold water, the contractions called *crimping* take place in about five minutes; but if the mass be large, it often requires thirty minutes to complete the process. It has been found that the muscles subjected to this process have both their absolute weight and specific gravity increased; whence it appears, that the water is absorbed, and condensation produced. It was also observed, that the effect was always greater in proportion to the voraciousness of the fish. The object, therefore, of *crimping* is to retard the natural stiffening of the muscles, and then, by the sudden application of cold water, to excite it in the greatest possible degree; by which means it acquires the natural firmness, and keeps longer. The operation certainly improves the flavour, as well as the

digestibility of the fish.   Turbot is an excellent article of
food; but it is usually rendered difficult of digestion by
the quantity of lobster or oyster sauce with which it is
eaten.   Sole is tender, and yet sufficiently firm; it is,
therefore, easy, of digestion, and affords proper nutriment
to delicate stomachs.   It is necessary to state, that every
part of the same fish is not equally digestible; and it
unfortunately happens, that those which are considered
the most delicious, are, at the same time, the most excep-
tionable: the pulpy gelatinous skin of the turbot, and the
glutinous parts about the head of the cod, are very apt to
disagree with invalids.   Salmon may, perhaps, be considered the most nutritive of our fish; but it is heating and
oily, and not very digestible: and persons, even with strong
stomachs, are frequently under the necessity of taking some
stimulant to assist its digestion.   The addition of lobster
sauce renders it still more unwholesome: the best condiment that can be used is vinegar.   As connected with the
time of spawning, the season of the year has the most
decided influence upon the quality of salmon.   It is in
the highest perfection, or *in season*, as it is termed, some-
time previous to its spawning; the flesh is then firm and
delicious; whereas, after this event, it is for some time
unfit for food.   This circumstance, however, is not sufficient to prevent those who have an opportunity, from
catching and eating the fish in that state; and the legis-
lature has accordingly found it necessary to fix the periods
at which salmon fishing is lawful.   In Ireland, where
there is great freedom used in killing salmon, during and
after the spawning season, the eating of the fish at such
times has been often found to be productive of disease;
and Dr. Walker has related a circumstance of the same
kind as having occurred in Scotland.   Salmon-trout is
not so rich and oily as the salmon; although, therefore, it
is less nutritive, it is, at the same time, less heating and
more digestible.   Eels are extremely objectionable, on

account of the large proportion of oil which they contain. I have witnessed several cases of indigestion and alimentary disturbance from their use. When eaten, they should always be qualified with vinegar. From these observations, the value of fish may be appreciated, and the qualities which entitle them to election easily understood. Firmness of texture, whiteness of muscle, and the absence of oiliness and viscidity, are the circumstances which render them acceptable to weak stomachs.

198. SHELL FISH have been greatly extolled by some physicians, as nutritive and easily-digestible articles of food. It will be necessary to examine this question, by the application of those principles which I have endeavoured to establish. Oysters, in my opinion, enjoy a reputation which they do not deserve : when eaten cold, they are frequently distressing to weak stomachs, and require the aid of pepper as a stimulant; and since they are usually swallowed without mastication, the stomach has an additional labour to perform, in order to reduce them into chyme. When cooked, they are still less digestible, on account of the change produced upon their albuminous principle. It is, however, certain, that they are nourishing, and contain a considerable quantity of nutritive matter in a small compass : but this latter circumstance affords another objection to their use. Certain it is, that oysters have occasionally produced injurious effects, which have been attributed to their having laid on coppery beds : but this idea is entirely unfounded, and arose merely from the green colour which they often acquire, the cause of which is now generally understood ; it is sometimes an operation of nature, but it is more generally produced by art, by placing them in a situation where there is a great deposit from the sea, consisting of the vegetating germs of marine *confervæ* and *fuci,* and which impart their colour to the oyster. For this object, the Dutch formerly carried oysters from our coasts, and depo-

sited them on their own.   Native oysters transported into
the Colchester beds, soon assume a green colour.   Where
this food has produced a fit of indigestion, it has evidently
arisen from the indigestible nature of the oyster, and the
state of the individual's stomach at the time; and had
such a person indulged, to the same amount, in any equally
indigestible aliment, there can be no doubt but that he
would have experienced similar effects.   Dr. Clarke has
related * some striking cases of convulsion, which occurred
to women after child-birth, in consequence of eating
oysters; the same effects might have supervened the ingestion of any food that is not easily digestible; for the
stomach of a woman at such a period, in consequence of
the irritable state of the nervous system, is easily disturbed
in its functions.   The oyster casts its spawn, which the
dredgers call the *spat*, in the month of May, after which
they are sick and unfit for food; but in June and July
they begin to mend, and in August they are perfectly
well.   We therefore see the cause of their going out of
season, and discover the origin of the old maxim, that an
oyster is never good except when there is an R in the
month.   Lobsters are certainly nutritive; but they are
exposed to the same objection, on the ground of indigestibility; and such has been their effect upon certain stomachs, as to have excited a suspicion of their containing
some poisonous principle: they have been known to occasion pain in the throat, and, besides eruptions upon the
skin, to extend their morbid influence to the production
of pain in the stomach, and affection of the joints.   As
found in the London market, they are generally under-
boiled, with a view to their better keeping; and in that
case they are highly indigestible.   The same observations
apply to the crab.   Shrimps are a species of sea crab,
which vary in their colour and size, and are considered

* Medical Transactions of the College of Physicians, vol. v.

easier of digestion than the preceding articles. The muscle is a species of bivalve which is more solid, and equally as indigestible as any animal of the same tribe. The common people consider them as poisonous, and in eating them, take out a part in which they suppose the poison principally to reside. This is a dark part, which is the heart, and is quite innocuous; the fact, however, is sufficient to prove, that this species of bivalve has been known to kill; but probably not more frequently than any other indigestible substance. Our annals abound with instances of the deleterious properties of melon, cucumbers, &c., and yet no one will contend that any poison, properly so called, resides in such vegetables. The peculiar cutaneous efflorescence which is produced by the imperfect digestion of shell fish, has been observed to occur more frequently in cases where the fish has been stale or tainted;* although it also happens where no such error can be suspected.

199. In eating some species of fish, as the pike, it is essential that the small bones should be carefully extracted; the swallowing of them is likely to irritate the alimentary membrane, and instances are recorded in which fistula has been thus produced.

---

* I am inclined to think that, under such circumstances, an *absolute* poison may be generated. Without this be granted, it will be impossible to explain many of the phenomena of fish-poison. Dr. Burrows has published a very striking case, in which two youths of the ages of nine and fourteen died, in consequence of eating about a dozen of small muscles, which they had picked from the side of a fishing-smack at Gravesend. The muscles were found to have been in a putrid state. In the *Gazette de Santé*, and in the works of Foderé and Behren, similar cases are recorded. Vancouver, in his voyage to the coast of America, relates, that several of his men were ill from eating some muscles which they had collected and roasted for breakfast; in an hour after which, they complained of numbness of the face and extremities, sickness, and giddiness. Three were more affected than the others, and one of them died.

200. It has been usual to attribute all the cutaneous affections which follow the liberal use of fish as depending upon the sympathy of the skin with the stomach. This, I believe, is, in general, the true explanation, since the effect is merely temporary; and when the process of digestion is finished, it departs. Its departure may even be hastened by the operation of an emetic removing the noxious aliment. At the same time, the fact must not be overlooked, that the oily principle, upon which depends the odour of certain fish, is absorbed from the alimentary canal, and carried into the blood; this is evident from the peculiar flavour of the flesh of certain birds who live upon fish: from the ready access which the hogs in Cornwall have to pilchards, the pork of that county is very commonly deteriorated by a fishy savour. It is also well known, that persons confined for any length of time to a diet of fish, secrete a sweat of a rancid smell. It is not, therefore, improbable, that certain cutaneous diseases may be produced, or at least aggravated, by such diet; and in hot climates this effect may be less questionable. The priests of Egypt may therefore have been prohibited from eating fish upon just principles, in order that the leprosy might be averted; and the great legislator of the Jews was, no doubt, influenced by some such belief, when he framed his celebrated prohibition.*

201. It is usual to add various condiments to fish, and many of them are doubtless thus rendered more digestible, by affording a necessary stimulus to the stomach: but rich sauces are ever to be avoided by the valetudinarian. Vinegar and salt, perhaps, form the best additions.

202. The mode of cooking fish is another circumstance of some importance; frying them in lard or oil is an objectionable process. In general, the process of boiling is best adapted to render them wholesome. Stewed fish,

* Leviticus, xi. 9—12.

with all the usual additions of glutinous and stimulant materials, are extremely injurious to dyspeptics. The objections which were urged against salted meats apply to salted fish ; they are, however, rendered less injurious by a plentiful admixture of potatoes : indeed, this esculent root, with perhaps the exception of parsnip, is the only vegetable that should accompany a meal of any species of fish : and it will be well for the invalid to abstain, upon such occasions, from fruit. Cullen says, that by way of experiment, he has taken apples after fish ; but he always found that his digestion was disturbed by them. Milk may be considered as another incompatible aliment ; the most serious diarrhœa has followed such a mixture.

BIRDS.

203. There exists a great variety in the qualities of the food which is furnished by this class of animals, with regard to nourishment, stimulus, and digestibility ; the whiter meat of domesticated birds, as the wings and breasts of chickens, contains less nutriment, and is less digestible, than that which is furnished by wild birds, as the partridge, &c.; but the former is, at the same time, less stimulant and heating than the latter. These are the circumstances which are to direct the medical practitioner in his opinion. No general rule for the choice of either species can be established : it must be determined by the particular condition of the patient, and the effect which the aliment is intended to produce. The same observation will apply to the flesh of quadrupeds ; that which is dark coloured, and contains a large proportion of fibrin, as venison, &c., is easily disposed of by the stomach, and a large quantity of highly-stimulating chyle is produced from it. The whiter meats are, on the contrary, detained longer in the stomach, and furnish a less stimulant chyle.

The former, therefore, will be more easily digested by weak persons, while the latter will frequently run into a state of acetous fermentation; but they may, nevertheless, be preferable on many occasions, inasmuch as they impart less stimulus to the general system. We see, therefore, the folly into which many popular writers have fallen, of stating such or such an article, as being wholesome or otherwise; *the wholesomeness of an aliment must depend upon its fitness to produce the particular effect which the case in question may require.* Van Swieten has justly said, that " to assert a thing to be wholesome, without a knowledge of the condition of the person for whom it is intended, is like a sailor pronouncing the wind to be fair, without knowing to what port the vessel is bound."

FARINACEOUS ALIMENTS.

204. We are principally indebted to the industry of man for this valuable addition to our *materia alimentaria.* The vegetables which yield it may be said to owe their nutritive qualities to cultivation. The art of feeding mankind on so small a grain as wheat, says Dr. Darwin, seems to have been discovered in Egypt, by the immortal name of Ceres; but it is probable, that it has risen to its present advanced state progressively, and is indebted to the labour of many generations for its perfection. The flour of wheat contains three distinct substances; a *mucilaginous saccharine matter, starch,* and a peculiar substance, possessing many of the properties of animal matter, termed *gluten.* It is to the quantity of this latter ingredient that wheat flour possesses so decided a superiority over that of barley, rye, or oats, for from these grains far less gluten can be extracted. It furnishes by far the best ingredient for making that important article of diet, BREAD; although it may also be made of all the various sorts of grain, as

well as of chestnuts, of several roots, and of the potatoe.
I shall first describe the nature of wheaten bread, and
then compare it with that produced from other substances.
The first process for rendering farinaceous seeds esculent,
is to grind them into powder, between mill-stones, which
Dr. Darwin aptly terms the " artificial teeth of society."
The *meal* thus produced is purified from the husk of the
seed, or *bran*, by the operation of sifting or *bolting;* and
it is then denominated *flour*. This, when mixed with
water or milk, undoubtedly possesses the power of nourishing the body; but it will evidently follow, from the observations which have been so frequently made in the progress
of this work, that in this raw state it would not be easily
digestible: it would clog the stomach, and oppose those
actions which are essential to chymification. The application, however, of heat, renders the compound more easy
to masticate as well as to digest ; whence we find, in the
earliest history, a reference to some process instituted for
the purpose of producing this change, although the discovery of the manufacture of bread, simple as it may
appear to us, was probably the work of ages. It has
been just stated, that wheaten flour is the best adapted
for making bread, that is to say, *loaf* bread ; this depends
upon the superior quantity of gluten which it contains,
and which operates in a manner to be presently explained.
The first stage of this process of purification consists in
mixing the flour with water, in order to form a paste, the
average proportion of which, is two parts of the latter to
three of the former ; but this will necessarily vary with
the age and quality of the flour : in general, the older and
the better the flour, the greater will be the quantity of
water required. This paste may be regarded as merely a
viscid and elastic tissue of gluten, the interstices of which
are filled with starch, albumen, and sugar. If, then, it
be allowed to remain for some time, its ingredients gradually re-act upon each other, the gluten probably per-

forming an important part; by its action on the sweet principle, a *fermentation* is established, and alcohol, carbonic acid, and lastly acetic acid, are evolved. If the paste be now baked, it forms a loaf full of eyes like our bread, but of a taste so sour and unpleasant that it cannot be eaten. If a portion of this old paste, or *leaven*, as it is called, be mixed with new-made paste, the fermentation commences more immediately, a quantity of carbonic acid is given off, but the gluten resists its disengagement, expands like a membrane, and forms a multitude of little cavities, which give lightness and sponginess to the mass. We easily, therefore, perceive why flour, deficient in the tenacity which gluten imparts to it, is incapable of making raised bread, notwithstanding the greatest activity may be given to the fermentative process by artificial additions. Where, however, *leaven* has been employed, the bread will be apt to be sour, in consequence of the great difficulty of so adjusting its proportion, that it shall not, by its excess, impart an unpleasant flavour, nor, by its deficiency, render the bread too compact and heavy. It is for such reasons that, in this country, we employ *barm ;* a ferment which collects on the surface of fermenting beer. It appears that we are indebted to the ancient Gauls for this practice. In Paris it was introduced about the end of the seventeenth century ; the faculty of medicine, however, declared it to be prejudicial to health, and it was long before the bakers could convince the public that bread baked with *barm* was superior to that with *leaven*. A great question arose among chemists, as to the nature of this *barm* that could produce such effects, and elaborate analyses were made, and theories deduced from their results ; but all these ingenious speculations fell to the ground, when it was found that *barm* dried, and made into balls, would answer every purpose : the bakers imported it in such a form from Picardy and Flanders, and when again moistened, it fermented bread as well as the recent substance. The presence, therefore, of carbonic acid, water, acetic acid, and alcohol, could not be essential, for these ingredients were separated by the process of its preparation. At length it was discovered, that gluten, mixed with a vegetable acid, produced all the desired effects ; and such is the nature of leaven, and such is the compound to which barm is indebted for its value as a panary ferment. After the dough has sufficiently fermented, and is properly raised, it is put into the oven previously heated, and allowed to remain till it is baked. The mean heat, as ascertained by Mr. Tillet, is 448°. When the bread is removed, it will be found to have lost about one-fifth of its weight, owing to the evaporation of water; but this proportion will be varied by the occurrence of numerous circumstances, which it is not easy to appreciate. Newly-baked bread has a peculiar odour as well as taste, which are lost by keeping: this shews, that some peculiar substance must have been formed during the operation, the nature of which is not understood. Bread differs very completely from the flour of which it is made, for none of the ingredients of the latter can be discovered in it; it is much more miscible with water than dough; and on this circumstance its good qualities, most probably, in a great measure depend. It is not easy to explain the chemical changes which have taken place. It appears certain, that a quantity of water, or its elements, is consolidated and combined with the flour ; the gluten, too, would seem to form a union with the starch and water, and thus to give rise to a compound, upon which the nutritive qualities of bread depend.

205. *Unleavened* bread consists of a mixture of meal and water, formed into a firm and tough cake, made as thin as possible, to favour its drying, and sometimes with the addition of butter, to render it more soluble, friable, and porous ; but it renders it sourer, and more apt to produce acidity on the stomach. Of the unleavened sorts of

bread, biscuit is by far the best ; and in all cases where
leavened or fermented bread does not agree, its use cannot
be too strongly advocated. I shall have occasion, hereafter, to relate cases in which the use of common bread
did not agree, and in which acidity of the stomach was
cured by the substitution of biscuit.

206. The different sorts of bread to be met with in
this country, may be considered under three classes ; viz.
whiten, wheaten, and *household.* In the first, all the *bran*
is separated ; in the second, only the coarser ; in the
third, none at all : so that *fine bread* is made only of flour,
wheaten bread of flour and a mixture of the finer bran,
and *household* of the whole substance of the grain, without
taking out either the coarse bran or fine flour. It is necessary for the medical practitioner to understand these
distinctions ; for it will be proved that an important
dietetic fact is connected with them. The tendency of
starch upon the bowels is astringent. Bread, therefore,
which is made of the whitest flour is apt to render them
costive ; but this is counteracted by the presence of *bran,*
the scales of which appear to exert a mechanical action
upon the intestines, and thus to excite them into action.
I have already stated, in the Pharmacologia, that there
are many bodies which have the power of thus acting
upon the inner coats of the intestinal canal, and of increasing its peristaltic motion ; and it is not improbable,
that the harsh and coarse texture which certain grasses
assume in moist situations, is a wise provision in nature
to furnish an increased stimulus to the intestines of the
animals who are destined to feed upon them, at a time
when their diminished nutritive qualities may render such
an effect salutary. The practical application of such views
is obvious ; and experience has sanctioned the propriety
of the practice that may be founded upon them. By
changing the quality of the bread, I have frequently succeeded in regulating the alvine discharges.

207. The French have many varieties of bread, in which eggs, milk, and butter, enter as ingredients. They are in the habit of adding ammonia to the dough; which, during its evaporation in the oven, raises it, and thus adds to its sponginess.

208. *Barley bread* has a sweetish but not unpleasant taste; it is, however, rather viscid, and is less nutritive as well as less digestible than wheaten bread. It is common to mix peas-meal witth the barley, which certainly improves the bread. *Rye bread* is of a dark-brown colour, and is apt to lie heavy on the stomach; it is also liable to create acescency and purging: but it appears to be highly nutritive. In some of the interior counties of England, where their bread is often manufactured from oatmeal, there is a mode of preparing the meal by making it sour; the bread, instead of being hard, is thus rendered of a soft texture, and from its moderate acidity is wholesome to strong persons: but invalids should, if possible, avoid it. In bread, however, this grain is more usually in an unfermented state, or it is made into flat, thin cakes, which are baked or roasted. The *bannock, clap-bread, bitchiness-bread,* and *riddle-cakes,* are the names which such productions have received. The *jannock* is oaten bread made into loaves. It is evident, from the health and vigour of the people who use this grain as a principal article of diet, that it must be very nutritive; but the stomach will require some discipline before it can digest it. In those unaccustomed to such food, it produces heartburn; and it is said to occasion, even in those with whom it agrees, cutaneous affections. In times of scarcity, potatoes have been made into bread; but they contain too much mucilage in proportion to their starch to afford a good article: the bread thus produced is heavy, and apt to crumble into powder; but such effects are obviated by mixing a certain quantity of wheat-flour with the potatoes. Rice will also serve the purpose of making very good bread;

but, like the potatoe, it requires the addition of some flour.
It is said by some, that bread, made of different kinds of
grain, is more wholesome than that made of only one sort,
as their qualities serve to correct one another. This is
certainly the case with that which is commonly called
brown bread, and which is made of a mixture of wheat
and rye flour; the former being of a more starchy nature
is apt to produce costiveness, while the latter often proves
too laxative: a due proportion of each, therefore, must
furnish a desirable compound.

209. The importance of bread, as an article of diet,
will be easily deduced from the principles upon which the
digestion of food in the stomach has been already explained. In addition to its nutritive qualities, it performs
a mechanical duty of some importance. It serves to
divide the food, and to impart a suitable bulk and consistence to it; it is therefore more necessary to conjoin it
with articles containing much aliment in a small space
than where the food is both bulky and nutritive. The
concentrated cookery of the French is rendered much more
wholesome from the large quantity of bread which that
people use at their meals. I know from personal experience how greatly this habit can correct the evil which
arises from rich soups and ragouts. If I eat a rich soup,
without a considerable quantity of stale bread, I inevitably
suffer from heartburn; but it never offends my stomach
when taken with such a precaution. Bread should never
be eaten new; in such a state it swells, like a sponge in
the stomach, and proves very indigestible. Care should
also be taken to obtain bread that has been duly baked.
Unless all its parts are intimately mixed, and the fixed air
expelled, it will be apt, in very small quantities, to produce
acescency and indigestion. After stating the advantages
of bread, it is necessary to make a few observations upon
the evils which it may occasionally produce; in certain
diseases it evidently produces a tendency to acidity: we

have daily instances of this fact in children, in whom acidity and much alimentary disturbance follow its use. In early life it is scarcely admissible, on account of the flatulence and costiveness which it produces ; and even at a more advanced period it gives children a pale counte-nance, and breeds worms. Shebbeare goes so far as to say, that the rickets are so common in France only because the quantity of bread given to children is excessive; which, by its acidity, destroys the calcareous substance of the bones, and reduces them to a state of cartilage. This is mere idle speculation, which is in direct variance with the received opinions upon the subject. Where acidity occurs, the bread should be toasted, or well-prepared biscuit sub-stituted. I shall have occasion to state, in a subsequent part of this work, that striking changes in the urinary deposits may be produced by suspending the use of bread, and giving biscuit in its place.

210. Bread has also been charged with producing evil consequences, from the presence of noxious principles, either naturally or artificially introduced into it. It will be necessary to direct some attention to these points. The presence of a peculiar poisonous principle, termed *ergot*, or *spurred rye*, has frequently proved a source of extensive disease: but as this subject has been ably treated in the various works on Toxicology, it will not be necessary to enter into its history on this occasion. Much has been said and written upon the subject of the adulteration of bread; but I am inclined to believe, that the evils arising from such a practice have been greatly exaggerated. It is certain, that the inferior kinds of flour will not make bread of sufficient whiteness to please the eye of the fasti-dious citizen, without the addition of a proportion of alum. It has been also found, that unless this salt be introduced into the flour, the loaves stick together in the oven, and will not afterwards separate from each other with that smooth surface which distinguishes the loaf of the baker.

This circumstance is probably owing to the action of the alum upon the mucilage of the flour, which it coagulates. It has been said, that the smallest quantity that can be employed for these purposes is from three to four ounces to two hundred and forty pounds of flour. It cannot be denied, that the introduction of a portion of alum into the human stomach, however small, may be prejudicial to the exercise of its functions, and particularly to dyspeptic invalids. It was found by Mr. E. Davy, of Cork, that bad flour may be made into tolerable bread by adding, to each pound, from twenty to forty grains of the common carbonate of magnesia. The operation of this substance in rendering the bread lighter, has not been satisfactorily explained; but, from my own experience of its effects, I apprehend that it neutralises an acid which is produced during the fermentation of inferior flour, and, becoming itself decomposed by the same action, gives out carbonic acid, and thus contributes to the sponginess of the loaf. The addition of salt greatly improves the digestibility of the bread, for reasons which have been already considered.

211. Besides bread, several other preparations are made by the solidification of flour, such as pudding, pancake, &c. The most digestible pudding is that made with bread, and boiled; flour or *batter* pudding is not so easily digested; and *suet* pudding is to be considered as the most mischievous to invalids in the whole catalogue. *Pancake* is objectionable, on account of the process of frying imparting a greasiness to which the dyspeptic stomach is not often reconciled. All pastry is an abomination: I verily believe, that one half, at least, of the cases of indigestion which occur after dinner parties may be traced to this cause.

212. Amongst the farinaceous aliments, the POTATOE holds a distinguished rank; but its digestibility greatly depends upon its kind, and the nature of the cookery to which it is subjected. That species which is known by

the name of *waxy* potatoe should be shunned by the dyspeptic, for it is so indigestible as to pass through the intestines in an unaltered state. The mealy potatoe, on the other hand, readily yields to the powers of the stomach, and affords a healthy nutriment; in some respects it supplies the place of bread, and should therefore be eaten with freedom whenever our food is concentrated. The process of mashing them certainly does not contribute to their digestibility; by such a process they are not so intimately mixed with the saliva : and when they are impregnated with the fat of roast meat, they should be studiously avoided. When boiled, care should be taken that they are not over-done; for in such a case, they are deprived of their nutritious qualities.

213. RICE is the general aliment of the people of the East, with whom it answers the same purposes as bread does with us. As it is not much disposed either to acescency or fermentation in the stomach, it furnishes a wholesome aliment when mixed with other food ; but, if taken in large quantities by itself, from its low degree of stimulant properties, it is apt to remain for a length of time in the stomach : this effect is greatly increased by protracted boiling. Where the stomach is in a state of relaxation and debility, it ought not to be taken without condiment; it is, for this reason, found necessary in the warmer climates to conjoin it with a considerable quantity of warm spices. There formerly existed a prejudice against its use, from a belief that it had a tendency to produce blindness. It is scarcely necessary to state, that such an idea has no foundation in truth. It is generally considered as astringent, and is, therefore, a popular remedy for diarrhœa; no astringent principle, however, has yet been discovered in its composition, and it is probable that it owes its virtues, on such occasions, to the mild and bland mucilage with which it abounds, shielding the intestines from acrimonious humours.

214. There are various other aliments in domestic use, which owe their qualities to starch, such as *sago, tapioca, arrow-root,* &c. From the mucilaginous form in which they are usually administered to invalids, they are not so digestible as is generally supposed; but where the stomach rejects more substantial viands, they are useful in themselves, as well as proper vehicles for the administration of vinous stimulants.

215. The leguminous productions, or *pulses,* may be considered as constituting the second division of farinaceous aliment. They differ little from grains, except in affording a more unctuous flour, which forms a milky solution with water, owing to the presence of an oily matter. Although they are highly nutritive, they are certainly more indigestible than seeds, and the bread they afford is apt to occasion flatulence, and to lie heavy on the stomach. The use, therefore, of this species of food is more circumscribed than that of the farinaceous seeds; it is principally confined to the lower classes, and to those possessing strong powers of digestion. In dyspeptic habits they ought on no account to be allowed; the symptoms of uneasiness which they produce in such persons is often alarming: flatulence and colic are the common consequences of their action. It has been said with some truth, that nature herself would seem to point out the necessity of mixing such food with other grains, for the soil becomes exhausted, unless it is alternately sown with grains and pulses; whereas, by such an alternation, the ground is preserved in a condition to afford a constant supply of nutriment. Pulses are employed in two very different states; in an early stage of their growth, when they are succulent; and when all their parts have reached maturity: in the former condition they are frequently acceptable to the stomach; but in the latter, they are only calculated for those who have strong digestive powers.

216. PEAS form a wholesome and light food, when

green and young, but when full grown and dry, they are very indigestible : in this latter state they contribute, in a remarkable degree, to the generation of gas in the intestines.   In the form of pudding they are, if possible, still more objectionable ; for, in addition to the bad qualities which depend upon their composition, are thus added those which arise from tenacity of texture.   Beans, like peas, are comparatively wholesome in their immature state. The Kidney-bean being eaten with its cod, is not so flatulent as other pulse : when well boiled, it is easy of digestion, but not very nutritive.

217. Nuts are generally supposed to have constituted the earliest food of mankind; and they still furnish, in some countries, a considerable source of food.   In this country they are principally known as an article of the dessert, although on some occasions they are eaten with our food ; they constitute a favourite accompaniment with turkey ; and I allude to this circumstance in order to guard dyspeptics against their use.   I was lately desired to see a person who, after such a repast, was seized with violent pain in the region of the duodenum, accompanied with distressing retching ; I instantly suspected the cause, and the appearance of the stools which were produced confirmed my supposition.   The chestnuts had swelled in the intestines, and produced an obstruction, probably at that part of the duodenum where it makes its exit through the ring of the mesentery ; or they might have lodged in the stomach, and produced an irritation upon the pylorus. With regard to composition, the chestnut may perhaps be considered as more nearly allied to the pulse than to the nut tribe, since it affords no oil by expression, and from its farinaceous qualities it may even be made into bread, although it is heavy and indigestible.   Its nutritive power must be considerable, since it forms the chief food of the lower orders in the plains of Lombardy ; and it has been conjectured, that it was the *acorn* so frequently mentioned

in ancient history and tradition. When eaten after dinner, an indulgence which can only be conceded to the most robust, it ought to be previously roasted; its digestibility is also increased by being kept for some time after it has been gathered. It is at the same time thus rendered more palatable, by the greater evolution of its saccharine principle.

218. The evils which may arise from the use of the chestnut are still more likely to occur after the ingestion of nuts, for they are more oily, as well as more viscid and glutinous: when eaten, they should always be accompanied with salt; but it would be wise to banish them entirely from our tables. It is much easier, as Dr. Johnson has said, to be abstinent than temperate; an aphorism which applies with peculiar force on this occasion; for there is a fascination in nuts which will lead most persons, who once begin to eat them, to take a quantity which the best-disposed stomach cannot bear with impunity. Hoffman observes, that dysenteric complaints are always more common in those years in which the harvest of nuts is plentiful; and there is not a physician in any practice who will be inclined to doubt his statement.

ESCULENT ROOTS.

219. These are of two kinds; those used as food, and those which principally answer the purposes of condiment or seasoning. Under the first division may be classed *turnips, carrots, parsnips, Jerusalem artichokes, radishes,* &c.; many of which, it will be seen, are seldom used solely for aliment, but are rather brought to our tables to qualify our animal food. Under the second division may be arranged *onions, garlic, horse-radish,* &c. It will be necessary to offer a few observations upon the qualities of these several roots.

220. The CARROT, from the quantity of saccharine

matter which it contains, is very nutritive and slightly
laxative; but it also possesses a large proportion of fibrous
matter, which in some stomachs prevents the digestion of
the root, and it passes through the bowels with but little
change : to obviate this effect, it ought to be very thoroughly boiled, and it should be eaten when young. It
appears to have been introduced by the Flemings, in the
reign of Elizabeth. The TURNIP is a very excellent vegetable, and, although it has the character of being flatulent,
is less liable to disagree with the stomach than the carrot;
it ought, however, to be well boiled, and the watery part
separated by pressure. Lord Townshend, secretary to
Charles I., was the person who introduced its use into
England; but it appears that the ancient Romans, in the
best period of their republic, lived much upon this root.
The PARSNIP is nutritive and digestible, although many
persons dislike it on account of its sweet flavour. The
JERUSALEM ARTICHOKE* is agreeable, but watery and
flatulent; it ought, therefore, never to be eaten without a
proper accompaniment of salt and pepper. RADISHES.
All the varieties of which have a pungent and acrid taste,
in consequence of a peculiar stimulating matter, which
resides in the cortical part of the root. They may be said
to contain little else than water, woody fibre, and acrid
matter, and cannot therefore be very nutritive ; they may
act as a stimulant and prove useful, but they ought
never to be eaten when old, as the quantity of inert matter
in such a condition is apt to disagree with the stomach.
From the consideration of radishes we pass, by an easy
transition, to that of onions, &c., for they appear to form

---

* The reader is aware, that this root of a species of sun-flower has no
botanical relation with the artichoke properly so called; its name is a
curious specimen of verbal corruption. The word *Jerusalem* is a corruption of *Gira-sole*, Turn Sun, or Heliotrope. It acquires the title of
artichoke from its supposed resemblance in flavour to that vegetable.

the connecting link between alimentary roots and those
used principally as condiment. The ONION, however,
although classed under this latter division, and must be
considered as valuable on account of its stimulating matter,
certainly contains a considerable proportion of nourishment.
This appears evident in their boiled state, by which process
their acrimony is exhaled, and a sweet mucilage separated.
Sir John Sinclair says, that it is a well-known fact, that a
Highlander, with a few raw onions in his pocket, and a
crust of bread, or some oat-cake, can travel to an almost
incredible extent, for two or three days together, without
any other sort of food. The French are fully aware of the
quantity of nourishment this plant affords; hence the soup
à l'oignon is considered by them as the best of all resto-
ratives. As a stimulant to the stomach and bowels, the
onion, in a raw state, is certainly of value, and this is
much enhanced by its diuretic qualities. The leek, garlic,
shallot, are of the same species, and possess qualities of
the same nature. HORSE-RADISH* is a warm and pungent root, and is highly valuable to the dyspeptic as a
stimulant; it is, perhaps, the best of all condiments for
the prevention of flatulence.

ESCULENT HERBS.

221. In this class are arranged the leaves and stalks
of such vegetables as are eaten at table in the form of
" greens and salads." Some ancient nations, we are told,
were accustomed to range over fields and woods in search

---

* The epithet *horse* is a Grecism : ιππος and βους, *i. e.* horse and bull,
when prefixed to any word, were used to express its comparative great-
ness. We have thus, *horse*-radish, or the *greater* radish ; horse-mint ;
bull-rush, &c. The great Dock is called *Hippo*-lapathum, and the horse
of Alexander, from the size of its head, *Bucephalus.*

of food, devouring, like animals, any wild herb they could
find likely to satisfy their hunger :

> " Quæ sol atque imbres dederant, quod terra creârat
> Sponte suâ, satis id placabat pectora donum."
>
> *Lucret.* lib. v.

Some herbs are still eaten in a raw state ; but they are far
less digestible than when cooked. During the heats of
summer they are refreshing, and are well calculated to
assuage that febrile state which full meals of animal food
are known to occasion. Of all these herbs, the WATER-
CRESS is the most beneficial; for, by operating in some
degree as an aromatic, it promotes digestion, and corrects
that tendency to flatulency which other raw vegetables are
apt to produce. According to Xenophon, the ancient
Persians lived upon water-cresses, which they considered
the most wholesome of vegetable productions. The LET-
TUCE is generally eaten with other herbs, in the form of a
salad, dressed with oil and vinegar. Some difference of
opinion has arisen with respect to the propriety of such
additions. Gosse, of Geneva, found that vinegar retarded
its solution in the stomach ; and oil has been stated by
others to render it less digestible. I have generally
found such condiments useful, and that dressed lettuce is
less likely to ferment in the stomach than that which is
eaten without them. Oil is known to have such an effect
in checking fermentation, and the vinegar is not found to
promote it. The lettuce contains a narcotic* principle;
and the effect of this is, in a great measure, obviated by a
vegetable acid. Those persons, therefore, who eat lettuce
with a view to obtain such effects, ought to take it without vinegar. Whatever difference of opinion may exist

---

* We are told that Galen, in the decline of life, suffered much from
morbid vigilance, until he had recourse to eating a lettuce every evening,
which cured him.

with regard to lettuce, there is none with regard to celery,
the digestibility of which is greatly increased by maceration in vinegar.   Cucumbers are by far the most unwholesome of all raw vegetables, and should be avoided as
poison by dyspeptics.   The vegetables which require to
be boiled are the different species and varieties of *colewort;*
the value of which does not depend so much upon their
nutritive quality as the tenderness of their texture.   On
this account, the cauliflower and brocoli are the species to
be preferred, particularly the younger sprigs of the former.
Of the kinds where the leaves only are employed, the
Savoy is of a sweeter and more tender texture than the
others, particularly its central and upper leaves.   The
Cabbage tribe appear to contain a peculiar essential oil,
whence the peculiar odour of cabbage water; this matter
is liable to produce offensive effects on the stomach.   The
vegetable should therefore be boiled in two successive
waters, in order to free it entirely from the noxious ingredient, and at the same time to render its texture soft and
digestible.   Asparagus is quickly dissolved in the stomach, and, when sufficiently boiled, is not disposed to
create flatulence or acidity : along with its mucilage it
frequently contains some sweetness, which affords a proof
of its nutritive quality.   From the peculiar odour which it
imparts to the urine of those who eat it, it appears to possess some active matter distinct from its mucilage; and it
is generally considered diuretic.   I have, however, prepared a strong infusion, as well as extract, from it, in
order to ascertain this point, and I have not been able to
discover any diuretic effects from its administration in
large doses.   Asparagus is only wholesome when in an
intermediate state, between root and plant.   When older
than this, it is remarkably acrid.

FRUITS.

222. These are generally regarded as articles rather of luxury than of food ; and were we to form our opinion of their value from their abuse, we should certainly be rather disposed to class them under the head of poisons than of aliments. Nothing can be more mischievous to the invalid than large quantities of apples, pears, and plums, in the form of dessert, after the stomach has been already loaded, and its good nature taxed to the utmost by its Epicurean master. But, when taken under other circumstances, they contribute to health, and appear to be providentially sent at a season when the body requires that cooling and antiseptic aliment which they are so well calculated to afford. It is not my intention to enter into a minute history of the several kinds ; but it will be useful to take a general view of the qualities which distinguish each division, and to state the circumstances which render them useful or objectionable.

223. Fruits may be arranged under the following heads : stone fruits, the apple species, small-seeded fruits, small berries, and farinaceous fruits.

224. The stone fruits have been denounced as the least digestible species by popular acclamation, and I am inclined to acquiesce in the truth of the assertion as a general proposition ; but much of the mischief that has been attributed to their use has arisen from the unripe state in which they were eaten. They are, however, certainly less digestible than other species, and more liable to undergo fermentation in the stomach. The hard pulp of certain plums remain also in the alimentary canal for a long time, and are frequently passed without having been materially changed. The ripe peach is the most delicious, as well as one of the most digestible of the stone fruits: the apricot

is equally wholesome; but the nectarine is liable to disagree
with some stomachs. Cherries are far less digestible:
their pulpy texture and skins are not easily disposed of
by the stomach; and as the sweetest species contain a
considerable excess of acid, they may be objectionable in
some cases, and desirable in others. The apple species is
not so dilute and watery as the foregoing fruits, and is
less apt to pass into a state of noxious fermentation; but
its texture is firmer, and on that account it is retained
longer in the stomach, and often proves indigestible. The
same observations apply to pears, except that their texture
being in general less firm, they are less objectionable.
The orange, when perfectly ripe, may be allowed to the
most fastidious dyspeptic; but the white, or inner skin,
should be scrupulously rejected, for it is not more digestible than leather. The small-seeded fruits are, by far, the
most wholesome. Of these, the ripe strawberry and rasp-
berry deserve the first-rank. The grape is also cooling
and antiseptic, but the husks and seeds should be rejected.
The gooseberry is less wholesome, on account of the indigestibility of the skin, which is too frequently swallowed.
The fruits to be classed under the head of small berries,
are the cranberry, the bilberry, and the red whortleberry.
These are seldom eaten, except when baked, and in that
state their acescency seldom proves injurious. The farinaceous fruits are universally unwholesome. The melon,
which is the principal one, is very apt to disagree with
weak stomachs, and should never be eaten after dinner,
without a plentiful supply of salt and pepper.

225. The most proper periods for indulgence in fruit
appear to be the morning and evening. On some occasions it may be taken with advantage at breakfast, or
three hours before dinner, and it affords a light and agreeable repast if taken an hour before bed-time; but these
regulations are to be influenced by circumstances which
no general rule can possibly embrace.

226. By cookery, fruit, otherwise unwholesome, may be converted into a safe and useful aliment. Apples, when baked, afford a pleasant repast; and from their laxative properties are well adapted to certain cases of dyspepsia. Fruit pies, if the pastry be entirely rejected, may be considered valuable articles of diet. Dried fruits are by no means so useful or safe as is generally imagined; the quantity of sugar which enters into their composition disposes them to fermentation.

227. Having offered some general rules with respect to the circumstances which render food salutary or noxious, and illustrated these principles by an examination of the several classes and species of aliments, it remains for me to say a few words upon the subject of their intermixture. I have already, in the introduction of this work (6), alluded to the mischief which arises from the too-prevailing fashion of introducing at our meals an almost indefinite succession of incompatible dishes. The stomach being distended with soup, the digestion of which, from the very nature of the operations which are necessary for its completion (81), would in itself be a sufficient labour for that organ, is next tempted with fish, rendered indigestible from its sauces; then with flesh and fowl; the vegetable world, as an intelligent reviewer* has observed, is ransacked from the *cryptogamia* upwards; and to this miscellaneous aggregate is added the pernicious pasticcios of the pastry-cook, and the complex combinations of the confectioner. All these evils, and many more, have those who move in the ordinary society of the present day to contend with. It is not to one or two good dishes, even abundantly indulged in, but to the overloading the stomach, that such strong objections are to be urged; nine persons in ten eat as much soup and fish as would amply suffice for a meal,

---

* See the review of my Pharmacologia, in the Journal of Science and the Arts, No. xxviii.

and as far as soup and fish are concerned, would rise from the table, not only satisfied but saturated. A new stimulus appears in the form of stewed beef, or *côtelettes à la suprême* : then comes a Bayonne or Westphalia ham, or a pickled tongue, or some analogous salted, but proportionately indigestible dish, and of each of these enough for a single meal. But this is not all; game follows; and to this again succeeds the sweets, and a quantity of cheese. The whole is crowned with a variety of flatulent fruits and indigestible knick-knacks, included under the name of dessert, in which we must not forget to notice a mountain of sponge cake.* Thus, then, it is, that the stomach is made to receive, not one full meal, but a succession of meals rapidly following each other, and vying in their miscellaneous and pernicious nature with the ingredients of Macbeth's caldron. Need the philosopher, then, any longer wonder at the increasing number and severity of dyspeptic complaints, with their long train of maladies, amongst the higher classes of society ? " *Innumerabiles morbos non miraberis, coquos numera.*" But it may be said, that this is a mere tirade against quantity ; against over-distention of the stomach ; that it argues nothing against variety of food, provided the sum of all the dishes does not exceed that which might be taken of any single one. Without availing myself of the argument so usually applied against plurality of food, that "it induces us to eat too much," I will meet the question upon fair grounds. It is evident that the different varieties of food require

---

* The custom of introducing cake after a rich entertainment is very ancient; but the cakes or "*mustacea*" of the Romans were very different compositions. They consisted of meal, aniseed, cummin, and several other aromatics : their object was to remove or prevent the indigestion which might occur after a feast. A cake was therefore constantly introduced, for such a purpose, after a marriage entertainment; and hence the origin of the " Bride Cake," which in modern times is an excellent invention for *producing*, instead of *curing*, indigestion.

very different exertions of the stomach for their digestion ; it may be that the gastric juice varies in composition, according to the specific nature of the stimulus which excites the vessels to secrete it ; but of this we are uncertain, nor is it essential to the argument : it is sufficient to know, that one species of food is passed into the duodenum in a chymified state in half the time which is required to effect the same change in another. Where, then, the stomach is charged with contents which do not harmonise with each other in this respect, we shall have the several parts of the mixed mass at the same time in different stages of digestion : one part will therefore be retained beyond the period destined for its expulsion, while another will be hurried forward before its change has been sufficiently completed. It is then highly expedient, particularly for those with weak stomachs, to eat but one species of food, so that it may be all digested and expelled at nearly the same period of time ; that when the duodenal digestion has been fully established, the operations of the stomach shall have ceased. I have, on a former occasion (98), insisted upon the importance of such a regulation, and it now leads me to make some remarks upon the periods best adapted for our meals, and upon the intervals which should be allowed between them.

ON THE PERIODS BEST ADAPTED FOR MEALS, AND ON THE INTERVALS WHICH SHOULD ELAPSE BETWEEN EACH.

228. It is not extraordinary that a discrepancy of opinion should exist upon a question which involves so many fluctuating circumstances. Controversy upon this, as upon many other subjects of diet, has engendered a disbelief in its importance ; and this scepticism has given a plausible pretext for indulgence on the one hand, and protracted fasting on the other, as the wishes or habits of mankind may have rendered most agreeable. It will therefore be difficult to convince the public of the necessity of those regulations which are so essential for the maintenance of health or for the cure of disease. We have been told that the best time for dining is, *" for a rich man, when he can get an appetite, and for a poor one, when he can get food."* But appetite in health is regulated by habit, and in disease it acts but as an imperfect monitor. Certain general principles, therefore, deduced from observation and experience, must be laid down for our guidance ; and these again in their application must be modified and adapted to the circumstances of every particular case.

229. All physicians concur in advocating the importance of regularity, both as it regards the number of meals and the periods at which they are taken. Those who have weak stomachs will, by such a system, not only digest more food, but will be less liable to those affections which arise from its imperfect assimilation, because, as Dr. Darwin has justly observed, they have, in such a case, both the stimulus of the aliment they take, and the periodical habit, to assist the process. The periods of hunger and

thirst are undoubtedly catenated with certain portions of time, or degrees of exhaustion, or other diurnal habits of life; and if the pain of hunger be not relieved by taking food at the usual time, it is liable to cease .till the next period of time or other habits recur. As these periods must vary in every individual, according to the powers of digestion, the degree of exercise taken, and the quality of the food, it frequently becomes necessary, in civilised life, to have recourse to intermediate meals, or *luncheons*, in order to support the powers of the stomach during the long interval which may occur between the conventional periods of repast. But to the dyspeptic patient, in search of health, such indulgencies are rarely to be permitted; unless, indeed, the circumstances under which he is placed leave him no option between long fasting and supplementary refection. I am more anxious to impress this precept upon the minds of invalids, as the anxiety of friends, and the popular errors which exist upon the subject of diet, are too apt to establish the mischievous belief, that " *a little and often*" will be more likely to restore the languid stomach to its healthy tone than moderate meals at more protracted intervals. The specious aphorism of Dr. Temple, that "the stomach of an invalid is like a schoolboy, always at mischief unless it be employed," has occasioned more dyspeptic disease than that respectable physician could ever have cured, had his practice been as successful as that of Æsculapius, and his life as long as that of an antediluvian. The theory upon which this objection rests has already been explained (98). The natural process of digestion is thus disturbed, and the healthy action of the stomach, as evinced by the return of moderate appetite, is entirely prevented. In answer to this reasoning, the patient will sometimes tell you, that frequent refreshment is essential to his comfort; that a sensation of faintness obliges him to fly to such a resource, in order to rescue himself from the distress which it occasions. This, in general, is an artificial want, created by habit, and must be cured by restoring the patient to regular meals, which is to be effected by gradually lengthening the intervals of eating. But, since no general rule is without its exceptions, so it may be observed, that there are cases of disease, in which the stomach is unable to bear any considerable quantity of aliment at one time, whence it becomes indispensable to repeat it at short intervals, in order to afford a sufficient proportion of nutriment; but as the patient acquires strength, such a system should be gradually abandoned.

230. But, though the advantage of regular meals at stated periods is desirable, it has been much disputed how many should be allowed in the day: some physicians have considered one, others two, three, or even five necessary. It is, perhaps, impossible to lay down a general rule that shall apply to every particular case. In some persons, the food rarely remains longer than three hours in the stomach; in others four, five, or even six hours. It is evident, that the repetition of the meals ought to be regulated by this circumstance, always avoiding the extremes of long fasting and repletion. Some nations have been satisfied with one meal a day; but the stomach would thus be oppressed with too large a quantity, and in the interval would suffer from the want of some nourishment in it. Such a plan, therefore, is neither calculated for persons of robust health, and who are engaged in much bodily exertion, and consequently require large supplies, nor for those of a weak habit, who are not able either to *take* or to *digest* such a quantity of aliment in a single meal as will be sufficient to supply the waste of the body during twenty-four hours. Celsus recommends the healthy to take food rather twice in the day than once; and Sanctorius says, that "the body becomes more heavy and uneasy after six pounds taken at one meal, than after eight taken at three; and that he who makes but one meal in

the day, let him eat much or little, is pursuing a system that must ultimately injure him." In my opinion, an invalid may safely take three frugal meals; or, on some occasions, even four, provided a certain quantity of exercise be insisted upon. It is reported, that when Alexander the Great turned away his cooks, on proceeding upon a march, he observed that he had no further occasion for such assistants, as he carried with him superior cooks;— a long morning's journey to create an appetite for his dinner, and a frugal dinner to give a relish to his supper.

231. I shall now consider the nature of the different meals, and the periods at which they can be taken with the greatest advantage ; repeating, however, that all general rules must be modified in their application according to particular circumstances.

232. BREAKFAST. This is, perhaps, the most natural, and not the least important of our meals ; for, since many hours must have intervened since the last meal, the stomach ought to be in a condition to receive a fresh supply of aliment. As all the food in the body has, during the night, been digested, we might presume, that a person in the morning ought to feel an appetite on rising. This, however, is not always the fact ; the gastric juice does not appear to be secreted in any quantity during sleep, while the muscular energies of the stomach, although invigorated by repose, are not immediately called into action : it is therefore advisable to allow an interval to pass before we commence the meal of breakfast. We seem to depart more from the custom of our hardy ancestors, with regard to breakfast, than any other meal. A maid of honour in the court of Elizabeth breakfasted upon beef, and drank ale after it ; while the sportsman, and even the day labourer of the present day frequently breakfast upon tea. The periods of their meals, however, were so generally different from those of modern times, that we cannot establish any useful comparison between them, without taking

into consideration the collateral circumstances which must have influenced their operation. The solidity of our breakfast should be regulated by the labour and exercise to be taken, and to the time of dining. Where the dinner hour is late, we should recommend a more nutritious meal, in order to supersede the necessity of *luncheon*, or what the French call *un déjeuner à la fourchette*. At the same time it must be remembered, that dyspeptic invalids are frequently incommoded by such a repast, if it be copious. Heartburn is a common effect of a heavy breakfast, especially if it be accompanied with much diluting liquid; and a question has consequently arisen as to the propriety of taking much fluid on these occasions. Some have recommended a *dry breakfast*, as peculiarly wholesome; and we have been told, that the celebrated Marcus Antoninus made a rule to eat a hard biscuit the moment he got up. I think it will not be difficult to shew the reasons why liquids are essentially necessary at this meal. To say nothing of the instinctive desire which we all feel for them, it is evident that there is a certain acrimony and rankness in all our secretions at that time; the breath has frequently a peculiar taint in the morning, which is not perceptible at subsequent periods of the day. This may be explained by the loss which the fluids of the body have sustained by perspiration, as well as by the quality of newly-elaborated matter introduced into the circulation during sleep. The experiments of Sanctorius have fully demonstrated the superior power of sleep in promoting the perspiration; insomuch, that a person sleeping healthfully, and without any unnatural means to promote it, will, in a given space of time, perspire insensibly twice as much as when awake. This fact is sufficient to prove the necessity of a liquid breakfast. Every physician, in the course of his practice, must have been consulted upon the propriety of taking meat, tea, or coffee, at breakfast. I shall, therefore, offer to the profession the results of my experience upon this subject; and I am encouraged in this duty by a conviction of the advantages which have arisen from my views of the question. A person who has not strong powers of digestion, is frequently distressed by the usual association of tea with bread and butter, or, what is more injurious, with hot buttered toast or muffin; the oily part of which is separated by the heat of the liquid, and remains in the stomach, producing, on its cardiac orifice, an irritation which produces the sensation of heartburn. On such occasions I always recommend dry toast, without any addition. New bread, or spongy rolls, should be carefully avoided. Tea, to many persons, is a beverage which contains too little nutriment: I have therefore found barley water, or a thin gruel, a very useful substitute. A gentleman some time since applied to me, in consequence of an acidity which constantly tormented him during the interval between breakfast and dinner, but at no other period of the day: he had tried the effects of milk, tea, coffee, and cocoa, but uniformly without success. I advised him to eat toasted bread, with a slice of the lean part of cold mutton, and to drink a large cup of warm barley water, for the purpose of dilution. Since the adoption of this plan he has entirely lost his complaint, and continues to enjoy his morning diversions without molestation. Hard eggs, although they require a long period for their digestion, are not generally offensive to the stomach; they may therefore be taken with propriety, whenever, from necessity or choice, the dinner is appointed at a late season.

233. Dinner. Among the Romans this was rather considered as a refreshment to prevent faintness, than as a meal to convey nourishment. It consisted principally of some light repast, without animal food or wine; but in modern times it is considered the principal meal, at which every species of luxurious gratification is indulged in. With regard to the proper period at which invalids should dine, physicians entertain but one opinion; it should be in the

middle of the day, or at about two or three o'clock. Sir
A. Carlisle has justly observed, that it is thus best adapted
to the decline of animal vigour, because it affords a timely
replenishment before the evening waning of the vital powers, and which naturally precedes the hour of rest; besides
which, the custom tends to prevent intemperance; while
late hours and a consequent state of exhaustion demand,
or seem to justify an excessive indulgence in strong drinks,
and in variety of food. The exact period, however, of dinner
must be directed by the physician with reference to the
necessary habits of his patient, the nature and time of his
breakfast, and, above all, to the rapidity or slowness of his
digestion. I will illustrate the importance of this precept
by the relation of a case which lately fell under my immediate notice and care. A gentleman, resident in a distant
part of the country, applied for my advice under the following circumstances. His health was generally good, but
he had lost all appetite for his dinner, and constantly experienced a sensation of weight and uneasiness after that
meal: I prescribed some laxative and bitter medicines,
and after a fortnight had elapsed I again saw him. He
then told me that he had not experienced the sensations
of which he had complained for some time; but that the
circumstance afforded him but little encouragement, as he
had uniformly found the same beneficial change whenever
he resided in London, which he was at a loss to explain,
as he took the same exercise in the country. I then in-
quired whether the hour at which he dined was the same
in both situations? when it appeared, that in the country
he dined at three, and in London at about six. I immediately suspected the origin of the complaint, and fortu-
nately touched the spring which unfolded the whole secret:
his digestion was remarkably slow, and the dinner in the
country was served up before the breakfast had been duly
digested. By my advice this evil was remedied; and he
has never since had any reason to complain of want of

appetite, or of the weight and oppression which had so long distressed him.

234. TEA. I have already stated my reasons (146) for considering this repast as salutary; and where it is practicable, exercise should follow it.

235. SUPPER. In the time of Elizabeth, the nobility and gentry were accustomed to dine at eleven, to sup between five and six, and to go to bed at ten. It is therefore evident, that any argument, in favour of this meal, founded upon the healthy condition of our ancestors, must be fallacious. By supper, in modern times, we understand a late meal just before bed-time. But as sleep is not favourable to every stage of digestion, it is very questionable whether retiring to rest with a full stomach can, under any circumstances, be salutary. During the first part of the process, or that of chymification, a person so situated may perhaps sleep quietly, unless indeed the morbid distension of the stomach should impede respiration, and occasion distress; but when the food has passed out of the stomach, and the processes of chylification and sanguification have been established, the natural propensity of the body is for activity, and the invalid awakes at this period, and remains in a feverish state for some hours. Upon this general principle, then, suppers are to be avoided; that is to say, *hearty* suppers, which require the active powers of the stomach for their digestion. The same objection cannot be urged against a light repast, which is generally useful to dyspeptics; and it has been truly and facetiously observed, that "some invalids need not put on their night-caps, if they do not first bribe their stomachs to good behaviour." An egg lightly boiled, or a piece of dry toast, with a small quantity of white wine negus, will often secure a tranquil night, which would otherwise be passed with restlessness. Amongst the intellectual part of the community, there has ever existed a strong predilection in favour of suppers; the labour of the

day has been performed; the hour is sacred to conviviality, and the period is one which is not likely to be interrupted by the calls of business. To those in health, such indulgencies may be occasionally allowed; but the physician should be cautious how he gives his sanction to their wholesomeness. The hilarity* which is felt at this period of the day must not be received as a signal for repairing to the banquet, but, as an indication of the sanguification of the previous meal (105).

On the Quantity of Food that ought to be taken at different Meals.

236. There is no circumstance connected with diet, which popular writers have raised into greater importance; and some medical practitioners have even deemed it necessary to direct that the quantity of food, appropriated to each meal, should be accurately estimated by the balance. Mr. Abernethy says, that " it would be well if the public would follow the advice of Mr. Addison, given in the Spectator, of reading the writings of L. Cornaro; who, having naturally a weak constitution, which he seemed to have ruined by intemperance, so that he was expected to die at the age of thirty-five, did at that period adopt a strict regimen, allowing himself only *twelve ounces* of food daily." When I see the habits of Cornaro so incessantly introduced as an example for imitation, and as the standard of dietetic perfection, I am really inclined to ask with Feyjoo,—did God create Lewis Cornaro to be a rule for all mankind in what they were to eat and drink? Nothing can be more absurd than to establish a rule of weight and measure upon such occasions. Individuals differ from each other so widely in their capacities for food, that to

---

* Breakfast has been considered the meal of *friendship;* Dinner that of *etiquette;* and Supper the *feast of wit.*

attempt the construction of a universal standard, is little less absurd than the practice of the philosophical tailors of Laputa, who wrought by mathematical calculation, and entertained a supreme contempt for those humble and illiterate fashioners who went to work by measuring the person of their customer; but Gulliver tells us, that the worst clothes he ever wore were constructed on abstract principles. How then, it may be asked, shall we be able to direct the proportion of food which it may be proper for an invalid to take? I shall answer this question in the words of Dr. Philip, whose opinion so exactly coincides with my own experience, that it would be difficult to discover a more appropriate manner of expressing it. "The dyspeptic should carefully attend to the first feeling of satiety. There is a moment when the relish given by the appetite ceases: a single mouthful taken after this, oppresses a weak stomach. If he eats slowly, and carefully attends to this feeling, he will never overload the stomach." But that such an indication may not deceive him, let him remember to *eat slowly*. This is an important condition; for when we eat too fast, we introduce a greater quantity of food in the stomach than the gastric juice can at once combine with; the consequence of which is, that hunger may continue for some time, after the stomach has received more than would be sufficient, under other circumstances, to induce satiety. The advantage of such a rule over every artificial method by weight and measure, must be obvious; for it will equally apply to every person, under whatever condition or circumstances he may be placed. If he be of sedentary habits, the feeling of satiety will be sooner induced; and if a concurrence of circumstances should have invigorated his digestive powers, he will find no difficulty in apportioning the increase of his food, so as to meet the exigencies of the occasion.

237. Although it must be admitted, that we all take more solid food in health than may be necessary for sup-

porting the body in its healthy state; yet it is important
to know, that too great a degree of abstinence will also
tend to weaken and distress both mind and body.   Men
who in the earlier ages, from a mistaken notion of religion,
confined their diet to a few figs, or a crust of bread and
water, were so many visionary enthusiasts; and the excessive abstinence to which some religious orders are subjected, has proved one of the greatest sources of modern
superstition.   The effects of feeding below the healthy
standard, are also obvious in the diseases of the poor and
ill-fed classes in many parts of England and Ireland; and
these are still more striking in those districts where the
food is chiefly or entirely vegetable, and therefore less
nutritious.   It is also well known, that the obstinate fasting
of maniacs often occasions a disease resembling the sea
scurvy.

238. Those who are induced from their situation in life
constantly to exceed the proper standard of diet, will preserve their health by occasionally abstaining from food, or
rather, by reducing the usual quantity, and living low, or
maigre, as the French call it.   A poached egg, or a basin
of broth, may on such occasions be substituted for the
grosser solids.   The advantage of such a practice has not
only been sanctioned by experience, but demonstrated by
experiment.   The history of the art of *"training"* will
furnish us with some curious facts upon this subject.   It
is well known that race-horses and fighting-cocks, as well
as men, cannot be preserved at their *athletic weight*, or at
the " top of their condition," for any length of time; and
that every attempt to force its continuance is followed by
disease.   A person, therefore, in robust health, should
diminish the proportion of his food, in order that he may
not attempt to force it beyond the athletic standard.   I
am particularly anxious to impress this important precept
upon the mind of the junior practitioner, as I have, in the
course of my professional experience, seen much mischief

arise from a neglect of it. A person after an attack of acute disease, when his appetite returns, is in the condition of a pugilist who is about to enter upon a system of *training;* with this difference, that he is more obnoxious to those evils which are likely to accrue from over-feeding. In a state of debility and emaciation, without any disease, with a voracious appetite, he is prompted to eat largely and frequently ; and he is exhorted by those not initiated in the mysteries of the medical art, to neglect no opportunity to " *get up his strength.*" The plan succeeds for a certain time, his strength increases daily, and all goes on well ; but, suddenly, his appetite fails, he becomes again unwell, and fever or some other mischief assails him. To the medical practitioner the cause of the relapse is obvious : he has attempted to force his strength too suddenly and violently beyond that athletic standard which corresponds with the vital condition of his constitution.

239. Any sudden transition from established habits, both with regard to the quantity and quality of food, is injudicious. This precept is the more important, as persons who have too freely indulged, and begin to feel the bad effects of their excesses, are disposed to alter their habits without the preliminary preparations. They leap at once from the situation which gives them pain or fills them with alarm, instead of quietly descending by the steps which would secure the safety of their retreat.

240. After long fasting, we ought also to be careful how far we indulge; this is a caution given to us by Avicenna, and practical physicians must be well aware of the penalty which attends a disobedience of it. When a famine occurred in the city of Bochara, those who had lived on roots and herbs, on their return to bread and flesh, filled themselves greedily, and died. But we need not search the annals of former times for an illustration : persons who have been enclosed in coal mines for several days without food, in consequence of the accidental falling

in of the surrounding strata, have not unfrequently lost
their lives from the too assiduous administration of food
after their extrication.   During the period of my student-
ship at Cambridge, Elizabeth Woodcock was buried under
the snow for the space of eight days : on her being found,
she was visited by those to whom so extraordinary an ad-
venture presented any interest ; and I can state, from my
personal knowledge of the fact, that she died in consequence of the large quantity of sustenance with which she
was supplied.   In the first volume of the Memoirs of the
Philosophical Society of Manchester, the case of a miner
is recorded, who after remaining for eight days without
food, was killed by being placed in a warm bed, and fed
with chicken broth.

241. The advantages which are produced by rendering
food grateful to invalids are so striking, that the most
digestible aliment, if it excite aversion, is more injurious
than that which, though in other respects objectionable,
gratifies the palate.   If feelings of disgust or aversion are
excited, the stomach will never act with healthy energy
on the ingesta ; and in cases of extreme dislike, they are
either returned, or they pass through the alimentary canal
almost unchanged.   On the other hand, the gratification
which attends a favourite meal is, in itself, a specific stimulus to the organs of digestion, especially in weak and
debilitated habits.   In the sixth edition of my Pharmacologia, I published a case which was related to me by
Dr. Merriman, highly illustrative of the powerful influence
of the mind upon these organs.   A lady of rank, labouring
under a severe menorrhagia, suffered with that irritable
and unrelenting state of stomach which so commonly
attends uterine affections, and to such a degree, that every
kind of aliment and medicine was alike rejected.   After
the total failure of the usual expedients to procure relief,
and the exhaustion of the resources of the regular practitioner, she applied to the celebrated Miss Prescott, and

was *magnetised* by the mysterious spells of this modern Circe. She immediately, to the astonishment of all her friends, ate a beef-steak, with a plentiful accompaniment of strong ale ; and she continued to repeat the meal every day, for six weeks, without the least inconvenience! But the disease itself, notwithstanding this treacherous amnesty of the stomach, continued with unabated violence, and shortly afterwards terminated her life. On the other hand, I could cite several cases to shew, that the most nutritive and digestible aliment may be rejected by the stomach, if any impression against its salubrity be produced. I remember a case in which, from some groundless suspicion, the idea of the food having been poisoned by copper was introduced, the persons at table became sick, one or two absolutely vomited, and the remainder complained of distress in the stomach and bowels.

Conduct to be pursued previous and subsequent to Meals.

242. As dietetic regulations are intended for the use of those who are either suffering under disease, or are compelled, from the precarious state of their health, to attend to every circumstance which may be likely to preserve it, it is scarcely necessary, in a professional work, to apologise for the introduction of advice which, to the robust and healthy, may appear frivolous and unnecessary. It is admitted, that nature never contemplated the necessity of confining men to a certain routine of habits ; nor did she contemplate, as far as we can learn, the existence of those diseases which may render such discipline necessary. We have in this place only to inquire into the habits which are most favourable or hostile to the process of digestion, and then to form a code for the direction of those who stand in need of such artificial assistance.

243. Exercise in the open air is essential to the well-being of every person ; but its degree must be regulated by the circumstances under which the individual is placed. The interval between breakfast and dinner is the period for active exertion; and the enjoyment of it, when not attended with severe fatigue, will strengthen and invigorate all the functions of the body. This, too, is the period when the mind may direct its energies with the greatest chance of success ; but it is important to remark, that *the valetudinarian and dyspeptic ought never to take his principal meal in a state of fatigue:* and yet I would ask, whether there is a habit more generally pursued, or more tenaciously defended? Ay, and defended too upon *prin ciple;*—the invalid merchant, the banker, the attorney, the government clerk, are all impressed with the same belief, that after the sedentary occupations of the day, to walk several miles to their villas, or to fatigue themselves with exercise before their dinner, or rather early supper, will sharpen their tardy stomachs, and invigorate their feeble organs of digestion. The consequence is obvious: instead of curing, such a practice is calculated to perpetuate, and even aggravate the malady under which they may suffer, by calling upon the powers of digestion at a period when the body is in a state of exhaustion from fatigue. Often have I, in the course of my practice in this town, cured the dyspeptic invalid, by merely pointing out the error of this prevailing opinion, and inducing him to abandon the mischievous habit which has been founded upon it. Do not let me be understood as decrying the use of moderate exercise before dinner; it is the *abuse* of it that I am anxious to prevent. No person should sit down to a full meal, unless he has had the opportunity of previously inhaling the open air, and taken a quantity of exercise, proportionate to his power of sustaining it without fatigue. Upon this point I agree with Mr. Abernethy, who says, " I do not allow the state of the weather to be

urged as an objection to the prosecution of measures so essential to health, since it is in the power of every one to protect himself from cold by clothing; and the exercise may be taken in a chamber with the windows thrown open, by walking actively backwards and forwards, as sailors do on shipboard." Horse exercise is undoubtedly salutary, but it should not supersede the necessity of walking; where the two modes can be conveniently combined, the greatest advantage will arise. I have heard that a physician of eminence has declared, that *"equitation is more beneficial to the horse than to his rider:"* my own experience on this subject will not allow me to concede to such a proposition; nor to that which maintains that *" riding is the best exercise for regaining health, and walking for retaining it."* It must be admitted, that the shaking which attends horse exercise, is salutary to the stomach and intestines; it is also less fatiguing to the inferior limbs; so that persons in a weak state can use it with less pain or difficulty. There is also another circumstance connected with this subject, upon which I am inclined to think that sufficient stress has not been laid, the rapidity with which we change the air. I am not aware that any theory has been proposed to explain the fact; but I am perfectly well satisfied, that rapid motion through the air is highly beneficial. As this is a gymnastic age, I may be allowed to offer some further observations upon the importance of exercising the body. The occupation of *digging* is more beneficial than is usually supposed; and to dyspeptic patients it proves useful, by the agitation thus occasioned in the abdominal region. Patients who have suffered from visceral congestion, have experienced the greatest benefit from it. I am induced to believe, that the general discontinuance of those manly exercises, which were so commonly resorted to by our ancestors in the metropolis, has contributed to multiply our catalogue of dyspeptic diseases; and I cannot but express my satisfaction

at the prospect of the establishment of a society for their
re-introduction. Stow, in his Survey of London, laments
the retrenchments of the grounds appropriated for pastimes,
which had begun to take place even in his day : what
would he say, could he now revisit the metropolis ?   It
has been truly observed, that had it not been for the effect
of bodily exercise, Cicero* would never have triumphed at
the bar, nor Julius Cæsar in the field.

244. One of the great evils arising from too sedentary
habits, is constipation of the bowels. This, however, may
to a certain degree be remedied, by standing for a certain
period ; and I have repeatedly known the greatest benefit
to arise from the student or clerk introducing a high desk
into his office, by which he is enabled to pursue his occupation in a standing posture.

245. I have already explained the necessity of exercise
at that period of the digestive process, when the chyle
enters the circulation (105); and it is, perhaps, not the
least of the evils which attend the modern fashion of late
dinners, that it should preclude the possibility of such a
regulation.   The utility of dancing may certainly be deduced from these views, and its propriety sanctioned on
just principles; but the lateness† of the hour at which
these recreations commence, and, what is worse, the excessive heat and ill-ventilation of the apartments in which
they are usually carried on, must counteract any benefit
which might otherwise attend an indulgence in them.   If
exercise be useful during the period of sanguification, pure
air is no less so ; and I shall take this opportunity of entering my protest against the introduction of *gas* into the
interior of our houses.   *Carburetted hydrogen* is a deadly
poison; and even in a state of great dilution, it is capable

---

* See Plutarch's Life of Cicero.

† In former times the ball commenced at six, and terminated at
eleven ; but now it begins at eleven and ends at six.

of exerting a very baneful effect upon the nervous system. I have been consulted on several occasions for pains in the head, nausea, and distressing languor, which evidently had been produced by the persons inhaling the unburnt *gas* in the boxes of our theatres. In order to afford additional support to the objections which I have urged upon this occasion, I shall quote an account of the effects produced upon Sir Humphry Davy by the inspiration of *carburetted hydrogen gas.* He introduced into a silk bag four quarts of this gas nearly pure, which had been carefully produced from the decomposition of water by charcoal, an hour before the experiment, and which had a very strong and disagreeable smell. " After a forced exhaustion of my lungs," says he, " the nose being accurately closed, I made three inspirations and expirations of the gas. The first inspiration produced a sort of numbness and loss of feeling in the chest and about the pectoral muscles. After the second inspiration, I lost all power of perceiving external things, and had no distinct sensation, except a terrible oppression on the chest. During the third expiration this feeling disappeared, I seemed sinking into annihilation, and had just power enough to drop the mouthpiece from my unclosed lips. A short interval must have elapsed, during which I respired common air, before the objects about me were distinguishable. On recollecting myself, I faintly articulated, ' *I do not think I shall die.*' Putting my finger on the wrist I found my pulse threadlike, and beating with excessive quickness. In less than a minute I was able to walk; and the painful oppression on the chest directed me to open air. After making a few steps, which carried me to the garden, my head became giddy, my knees trembled, and I had just sufficient voluntary power to throw myself on the grass. Here the painful feeling of the chest increased with such violence as to threaten suffocation. At this moment, I asked for some

nitrous oxide.* Mr. Dwyer brought me a mixture of
oxygen and nitrous oxide, which I breathed for a minute,
and *believed* myself relieved. In five minutes, the painful
feelings began gradually to diminish. In an hour they
had nearly disappeared, and I felt only excessive weakness
and a slight swimming of the head. My voice was very
feeble and indistinct: this was at two o'clock in the afternoon. I afterwards walked slowly for about half an hour;
and on my return was so much stronger and better, as to
believe that the effects of the gas had disappeared, though
my pulse was 120, and very feeble. I continued without
pain for nearly three quarters of an hour, when the giddiness returned with such violence as to oblige me to lie on
the bed; it was accompanied with nausea, loss of memory,
and deficient sensation. In about an hour and half the
giddiness went off, and was succeeded by an excruciating
pain in the forehead, and between the eyes, with transient
pains in the chest and extremities. Towards night these
affections gradually diminished; at ten, no disagreeable
feeling except weakness remained. I slept sound; and
awoke in the morning very feeble and very hungry. I
have," adds Sir H. Davy, " been minute in the account
of this experiment; because it proves, that carburetted
hydrogen acts as a *sedative, i. e.* that it produces diminution
of vital action, and debility without previously exciting.
There is every reason to believe, that if I had taken four
or five inspirations, instead of three, they would have destroyed life immediately, without producing any painful
sensation."† After this proof of the poisonous nature of
carburetted hydrogen,—after the cases of sickness and
headach which have occurred, in consequence of its

* Sir H. Davy had previously inspired this gas, and found it capable
of producing an excitement resembling that of incipient intoxication.

† " Researches, Chemical and Philosophical, chiefly concerning
Nitrous Oxide, and its Respiration, by Humphry Davy."

inhalation at the theatre, am I not borne out in my opinion,
that *its introduction into our apartments is fraught with
danger?*

246. Sleeping after dinner is a practice of very questionable propriety ; it is true, that the inhabitants of many
southern climates indulge it with impunity : but it does
not appear essential in our country, where animal food is
used in such considerable quantities. In states of disease
it may occasionally be useful, and the recumbent posture
may expedite the passage of the aliment out of the stomach into the intestines; but the person who lies down
for the accomplishment of such an object, should be careful to remove all ligatures from his body.

On the Influence of different Aliments in
Modifying the Appearances of the Discharges of the Body.

247. The external characters of the feculent discharges
of the body, may be said to announce the healthy or diseased
state of the digestive functions, with as much certainty as
the pulse does that of the sanguiferous system. But, in
order that we may deduce safe conclusions from such data,
we must be acquainted with the nature and extent of the
changes which are produced on these discharges by the
operation of different aliments and medicines. The air
has also the effect of changing the colour of the fæces ;
they should therefore be examined before such an alteration is likely to be produced. This observation applies
with great force to the stools of infants, which, although
perfectly yellow when voided, speedily assume a green
appearance; a fact which would seem to arise from the
spontaneous decomposition of the bile.

248. Certain green vegetables, especially spinach, impart to the fæces a green hue, which may be mistaken

for vitiated bile.   Beet-root will also give a colour to the
alimentary discharge, which it is necessary to distinguish.
Persons who take a considerable quantity of milk, will pass
pale-coloured evacuations, as if the bile were imperfectly
secreted.   Where the aliment has been of a very complicated description, the fæces will generally assume a crude
and diversified character, owing, probably, to the several
parts not having undergone the same degree of digestion,
as already explained (227).   Where much stimulant drink
has been used, and the person has been subjected to long
fasting, or much labour, or has perspired profusely, the
fæces acquire a hardened character.   It is essential for
the practitioner to know, that certain parts, both of animal
and vegetable substances, pass through the body without
undergoing any change : this is the case with the skin and
seeds of fruits, &c.   Cheese is also very apt to pass in an
undigested state.   Dr. Marcet records an instance of this
kind, in which the substance was at first mistaken for an
intestinal concretion ; but it proved to be either a piece of
cheese formed into a ball by the action of the intestines,
or a portion of caseous matter actually formed in the intestines, from milk taken as nourishment by the patient,
and coagulated by the gastric juices into an undigestible
mass.   This latter supposition is the more probable, as
Dr. Wollaston, a few years afterwards, had several concretions of the same kind brought to him for examination
by a medical practitioner, and which proved of the same
nature, and had been discharged by a patient whilst using
a milk diet.   It has also been stated by Dr. Marcet, that
concretions of oat seeds are not unusually passed by the
inhabitants of Scotland and Lancashire, where the oat-
cake is in common use as an article of food amongst the
lower classes.   The spawn of lobsters, a very indigestible
substance, has also occasioned similar deception.   Magnesia, when repeatedly taken, will, by the assistance of a

little animal mucus, become consolidated into masses of formidable magnitude. Mr. E. Brande has recorded an interesting case of this kind in the first volume of the Journal of the Royal Institution. The influence produced by certain medicines upon the colour of the fœces, is equally striking; iron has the property of tinging them black, and magnesia, of giving a white appearance. We see, therefore, the importance of attending to such circumstances, where it is an object to ascertain the state of the biliary secretion from the colour of the stools; and it would be judicious, on such occasions, to restrict patients to a diet that is not likely to colour the fœces.

249. I have now brought to a conclusion the history of Alimentary Substances. It will be readily perceived, that the terms *digestible* and *indigestible*, as applied to particular species of food, are but relative in their import, depending upon circumstances which I have endeavoured to investigate : with what degree of success I have performed this task, it will be for the public to decide; but I may be allowed to observe, that the importance which I have bestowed upon some, perhaps, apparently trivial circumstances, has arisen from a belief, founded on practical grounds, in the influence which they exert on the human body; while, if I have passed over others with less notice than they may appear to deserve, it has arisen from a conviction that they have either been overrated in importance, by those writers who have indulged in discussions upon them, or are so involved in doubt and uncertainty, that I have despaired in throwing any additional light upon their nature and bearings. The theory of Digestion, and the history of Alimentary Substances, are so intimately connected with the diseases to which our organs are exposed, that without a thorough knowledge of the former, we cannot expect to understand the phenomena of the latter; nor to establish a rational and suc-

cessful system of treatment for the prevention and cure of Dyspepsia. I shall now proceed to the third division of the work, which will embrace the history of INDI- GESTION in all its forms and stages; in which I shall hope to turn the principles, already developed, to a prac- tical advantage.

PART III.

OF

INDIGESTION.

PART III.

OF

INDIGESTION.

250. It has been already observed (8) that authors have differed in their acceptation of the term DIGESTION. Some regarding it as merely denoting that preparatory process which the food undergoes in the stomach; while others have received it in a more extensive latitude, as comprehending the whole of that elaborate and complicated series of actions, by which nature converts bread into blood. We cannot, therefore, be surprised to find that pathologists should as widely have differed in their definition of the disease termed DYSPEPSIA, or INDIGESTION. Notwithstanding the distinction which Dr. Philip is disposed to establish between these terms, by considering "*Dyspepsia*" as expressing a disease much less varied, and of much less extent, than that which he comprehends under the denomination of "*Indigestion*," I am still disposed to regard them as synonymous; and when they occur in the following pages, I must beg the reader to receive them with that impression. The term *Indigestion* is evidently nothing more than a literal English translation of the Greek compound *Dyspepsia*.

251. I define IN DIGESTION to be *a primary disease, in which one or more of the several processes by which food is converted into blood, are imperfectly or improperly performed, in consequence either of functional. aberration, or organic lesion.* This definition may, perhaps, be opposed, on the ground of its too comprehensive signification; but I may observe, that however extensive may be the series of symptoms which are thus included under one general head, they will afford, when viewed collectively, sufficient evidence of their relation with the digestive process; although, on a loose and hasty observation, they may not present any general principle of dependency and connection: if they appear disunited, let the practitioner suspect that he has never viewed them with sufficient reference to that physiological harmony which subsists between the organs in which they arise. Acidity of stomach and urinary depositions are equally indicative of deranged digestion; but the mind that is not acquainted with the relations of the stomach and kidneys, or with the connection which subsists between the formation of perfect chyle and the discharge of natural urine, will not be disposed to arrange symptoms, so apparently remote in their alliance, under one common head. There are many sympathies subsisting between different functions which are not perceptible as long as the general balance of health is preserved: this is remarkably the case with the skin and stomach; but the moment this healthy equilibrium is destroyed, the sympathies become apparent. The physiologist, therefore, without an acquaintance with the body in its morbid states, must remain ignorant of some of the more important circumstances of the animal economy. The same reasoning applies to the study of natural philosophy: the discovery of the existence of an electric fluid could never have been made, had the natural conditions of matter, with regard to this agent, remained unchanged; the basis of all chemical research is founded

upon the same principle; decomposition, and the deve-
lopement of the elements of bodies, are effected by over-
turning the affinities by which they are naturally combined. These observations are introduced in order to
warn the practitioner not to deduce any conclusion
against the existence of certain sympathies, on the ground
of their not being apparent in a state of health. In a
practical point of view, I consider the classifications of
the nosologist as of very little utility; they have no solid
foundation in nature, but are entirely the work of human
reason; artificial contrivances, for the purpose of assisting
us in the acquirement and retention of knowledge. Such
an avowal will sufficiently explain the motive which has
induced me to throw off the trammels to which I might
have been expected to conform.

252. From the universal sympathy which the stomach
entertains for every part of the living body, its functions
may become impeded or perverted from the existence of
diseases which originate in organs with which it has no
immediate connection; an affection of the head, or even a
disease in the urethra, may create sickness, loss of appetite, or a suspension in the digestive process; but such
phenomena are not to be confounded with the primary
symptoms of Dyspepsia; they are affections of sympathy
or induction, and will require very different treatment.
In distinguishing between such effects, consists the skill
of the practitioner; and it requires a comprehension of
mind, a freedom from prejudice, a clearness of judgment,
and a patience of minute enquiry, that do not fall to the
lot of every member of our profession. I am strongly
inclined to think that physicians of the present day are
too apt to accuse the alimentary functions of offences
which should be charged on other organs. It is, perhaps, natural in those who have devoted much time and
attention to one particular subject, to fall into an error of

this kind ; they have a favourite child of their own to support, and they prefer it with the blind partiality of a parent. As connected with this opinion, I beg to direct the reader's attention to the first case which I have introduced, in my " practical illustrations," at the end of the present volume.

I. Imperfect Chymification.

253. The symptoms which arise from the food undergoing its appointed changes in the stomach with difficulty, or in an imperfect manner, are generally those which first indicate the approach of indigestion, and frequently recur at intervals, for a considerable period, without occasioning any constitutional disturbance, or even a degree of local distress sufficient to awaken the alarm of the patient. In some cases, indeed, they are only produced by the use of particular aliments, or under the operation of peculiar circumstances ; but in others, they follow the ingestion of every species of food, although their violence is usually influenced by the quality and quantity of the meal. In this latter case, a morbid state of the stomach exists, which ought to be remedied without delay. In investigating the circumstances of an indigestion, produced only by some particular aliment, we shall soon discover whether it is to be attributed to a peculiar idiosyncrasy of the stomach, which cannot be said to amount to disease, or to a debilitated condition of that organ, which renders it unable to digest any food that requires considerable powers for its chymification. The mucous membranes of the stomachs of certain persons, appear to be irritated by particular aliments, as the skin is known to be by particular coverings : I am acquainted with a person who can never wear cotton stockings without suffering from considerable cutaneous irritation ; and I also know a

gentleman who is incapable of eating the smallest quantity of mackarel without experiencing uneasiness in the stomach, and yet he digests every other species of food with facility : this is not disease, but idiosyncrasy, and it is very essential to distinguish them from each other. If, on the other hand, a person informs me that, as long as he lives upon mutton, or beef, that his digestion goes on well, but that if he eats pork, veal, or fried meat, he suffers from heartburn, and other unpleasant feelings in his stomach, I deduce a different conclusion, and infer that his general powers of digestion are feeble, and easily depressed ; and that he is consequently unable to convert into healthy chyme those aliments which require a higher degree of exertion.

254. There is no fact better understood, than that the living principle of our organs possesses the power of preventing the chemical changes to which their contents would, under other circumstances, be exposed. The blood does not coagulate or putrefy in the vessels ; the urine does not undergo decomposition in the healthy bladder ; nor does the food ferment in the stomach, unless that organ be in a state of disease ; but if its vital powers fail, the chemical affinities gain the ascendency, and, after a certain interval, various symptoms arise, which clearly evince the change which has been produced. This is the philosophy of an ordinary attack of indigestion, when, either from the quantity or quality of the food, the stomach is inadequate to perform its necessary duties. An uneasiness and sensation of weight and distention is experienced in the region of the stomach, acidity prevails, and eructations of disengaged air distress the patient; a sensation of nausea is felt, arising from an effort of the stomach to eject that which it is unable to digest. Chilliness is perceived, and a general lassitude arises from the sympathy which is produced on the nervous and sangui-

ferous systems. These effects are felt particularly towards the end of chymification, and, after a certain
period, pass off, and the remaining parts of the process
are apparently conducted with regularity. But this is a
statement of the symptoms which attend a casual fit of
dyspepsia, as it may occur to persons in health, from the
influence of various circumstances, such as an overloaded
stomach, indigestible food, a too hearty meal after long
fasting or fatigue, obstructed bowels, or any other cause
which may occasion a temporary debility of the stomach.
It is only necessary, in such a case, to avoid in future the
exciting causes, and to clear the bowels of any superfluous and crude matter which may be supposed to lodge
in them. But lightly as we may, in general, treat a
casual indigestion of this kind, cases are on record which
should awaken us to a sense of its possible mischief,
especially if the subject of it be a person advanced in
life. If a patient retires to rest before the stomach is
relieved from its load, he may pass into a comatose state,
accompanied with apoplectic stertor, from which it is not
unfrequently difficult to rouse him; and which arises
from the sympathy of the brain with the oppressed
stomach. It is of great importance to distinguish such
an affection from genuine apoplexy, since, if the stomach
be not relieved, the stupor increases, and the patient is
lost. We should carefully examine the epigastrium, in
order to ascertain whether any considerable fulness can
be felt in that region, and enquire into the history of the
patient: if he can be awakened, no time should be lost in
administering an emetic, and it will be a safe practice to
abstract a quantity of blood from the arm, which will
have the additional advantage of accelerating the operation of any medicine that may have been administered for
his relief.

255. It must, however, be allowed that such attacks

from an overloaded stomach are not frequent; and are unlikely to occur, except the muscular powers of that viscus be so impaired as to prevent the usual efforts which nature employs to throw off an unmanageable burthen.

256. Should indigestion in the stomach continue to recur, the paroxysm will assume a more troublesome character; its symptoms will increase in number and extent, and the mischief will speedily involve other functions: but before I proceed to follow the course which it usually runs, it will be useful to examine the causes to which the origin of the disease in the stomach is to be attributed.

257. It has been stated (65) that, in every change which the aliment undergoes, we shall discover the combined operation of mechanical and chemical agents: when the food, therefore, is introduced into the stomach, it owes its conversion into chyme to such combined actions, viz. the chemical power of the gastric juice, and the mechanical movements of the stomach. It is to the failure or imperfect operation of the one or the other of these necessary actions that indigestion is to be attributed. However perfectly the gastric juice may be secreted, if the mass be not sufficiently *churned* in the stomach, it cannot become perfect chyme; and the most active motions of the stomach will not compensate for a deficiency in the alimentary solvent. It signifies very little whether the paucity of the gastric liquor be absolute or relative; that is to say, whether it be originally secreted in less than a natural proportion, or the quantity of food taken be so great that the usual proportion of the solvent is insufficient for its solution; in either case, an indigestion must follow; although there appears to exist an accommodating power in the *healthy* stomach, which enables it to regulate its supply according to the call which may be made for it.

258. The quality and quantity of the gastric fluid,

secreted by the stomach, may be influenced by causes immediately acting upon that organ, or by those which affect it through the medium of sympathy. Under the first class of causes may be noticed those which produce a direct influence upon the nerves of the stomach, without whose healthy action no secreting surface can perform its functions with regularity. Amongst these, the injudicious ingestion of narcotic substances, or of alcohol, deserve a distinguished notice. The languor arising from inanition also brings on what Mr. Abernethy calls a " discontented state of the stomach;" in which case, the gastric juice is not secreted in a healthy manner. But the causes which act locally on the secreting powers of the stomach are few in number, and perhaps small in importance, when compared with those which act through the medium of sympathy. During the periods at which the posterior stages of digestion are performed, the healthy secretion of gastric juice is not easily excited; and if, therefore, food be presented at these times, it will be apt to occasion indigestion. An overloaded state of the bowels will be attended with the same consequence ; exercise, when accompanied with fatigue, or indolence, may, by producing general debility, occasion a corresponding state of collapse in the stomach. Passions of the mind, fear, anxiety, and rage, are also well known to affect the nervous system, and through that medium, the stomach; and so immediately are its consequences experienced, that a person receiving unpleasant intelligence at the hour of a repast, is incapable of eating a morsel, whatever might have been his appetite before such a communication.

> ———— " Read o'er this ;
> And after this ; and then to breakfast
> *With what appetite* you have."

259. The sympathy subsisting between the skin is another source, and often an unexpected cause of gastric

debility. If the cutaneous vessels be unusually excited, and this excitation be continued for any length of time, they will at length fall into a state of indirect debility, whence a sense of faintness, loss of appetite, and inability of digesting solid food, will be experienced. This fact explains the diminished appetite of which persons complain in hot weather, and that universal custom in tropical climates of combining the food with large quantities of aromatic stimulants. One of the most striking instances indicative of this consent between the skin and stomach, is, where cold or wet is applied to the lower extremities, exciting pain in that organ and indigestion. Violent spasms, and in persons predisposed to gout, an attack of that disease in the stomach, have been occasioned by remaining for some time with the feet thoroughly wet. The custom of pouring spirit into the shoes or boots upon such occasions, from the mistaken idea of counteracting the evil, increases the mischief, from the additional cold produced by its evaporation. The first object, under such circumstances, is to prevent evaporation; and the chance of taking cold is greatly diminished, if not entirely prevented, by covering the wet clothes with some dry garment. It has been said, and perhaps with some reason, that the thin shoes and light dress render delicate females, notwithstanding their temperance, more subject to the whole tribe of dyspeptic complaints, particularly flatulence and want of appetite.

260. As the skin acts upon the stomach, so does the stomach, in its turn, re-act upon the skin; for all sympathies are reciprocal. A physician who is conversant with affections of the stomach, well knows how to appreciate the indications which the appearance of the countenance affords; there is a peculiar pallor and relaxed condition of the skin, which is truly indicative of a deranged state of the digestive organs, and which gradually disappears under a successful treatment. The want of appetite for

breakfast, which is complained of by invalids, is frequently
to be attributed, amongst other causes, to the atony produced on the surface of the body, and consequently on
the stomach, by sympathy, by the relaxing influence of a
warm bed; and hence arises the utility of restoring a
reaction, by fresh air and exercise, before we attempt to
sit down to our morning repast.   The warm bath, if not
at too high a temperature, or indulged in for such a length
of time as to induce indirect debility, will be found, by its
stimulant operation on the skin, to place the stomach in a
condition to digest the dinner when employed a few hours
before that meal.   I shall have to refer to these facts
when I come to consider the modes of curing indigestion.

261. The influence of a healthy condition of the digestive organs upon the skin, is so well understood by those
that direct the art of training, that the clearness of the
complexion is considered the best criterion of a man
being in good condition, to which is added the appearance
of the under-lip, " which is plump and rosy, in proportion
to the health of the constitution."

262. The stomach also sympathises, in a remarkable
degree, with the urinary organs; nephritic complaints are
invariably attended with nausea.   I lately had a very
troublesome case of dyspepsia under my care, which was
aggravated, if not originally produced, by a troublesome
stricture in the urethra, which kept up a constant irritation.

263. I have next to consider the causes which may
operate in depressing or paralysing the muscular powers
of the stomach, by which the mechanical process, essential to chymification, is imperfectly performed.   Of these,
undue distention is perhaps the most common, and, at
the same time, the most powerful.   This may be proved,
not only from ample observation on the stomach, but by
the analogy of other cavities : if the bladder be distended
for some time with urine, its muscular powers are para-

lysed; it has often happened that where a person has, from necessity, retained his urine for a considerable time, on attempting to void it, he has found himself incapable of expelling a single drop, although the bladder has been ready to burst from over-distention. The same fact occurs with respect to the rectum: if this observation be applied to the stomach, we shall easily perceive why, in an over-distended state of that viscus, vomiting can scarcely be produced by the most violent emetic; and we shall readily understand from the same train of argument, how greatly the muscular fibres may become *permanently* debilitated by the repetition of such an excess. This over-distention is particularly apt to occur in cases where the food has a tendency to swell, from the heat and moisture of the stomach; for a person may not be aware of the quantity he has taken from any sensation of fulness at the time he ceases to eat, and yet, in the space of an hour, he may experience the greatest uneasiness from such a cause. This generally happens where much new bread has been taken; nuts have also this property in a remarkable degree, and ought, for such a reason, to be prohibited, where such an effect is to be apprehended. A draught of soda water, or any beverage which contains fixed air, may be visited with the same penalty. There are certain postures of the body, which, by preventing the necessary egress of the contents of the stomach, favour an accumulation in its cavity; this occurs in the occupation of the shoemaker, tailor, engraver, from stooping on the last, or desk, by which their thoracic and abdominal viscera are compressed together for many hours; the margin of their ribs is pressed upwards, so as to force the stomach against the diaphragm, and to impede the passage through the pylorus: it is evident, that if such a habit be continued after a full meal, that all the train of dyspeptic terrors must be produced; and we have all witnessed too many practical illustrations of the fact,

to require farther evidence of its truth. The profession
is much indebted to Dr. W. Philip, for having proved
by experiments, related in his Inquiry into the Laws of
the Vital Functions, that the muscular fibre, though
independent of the nervous system, may, in every instance, be influenced through it; from which it follows,
as a corollary, that the muscular fibres of the stomach
may not only be affected by causes acting directly on
them, but *by such as act through the medium of the nerves.*
Hence, the presence of offensive matter in the stomach,
whether arising from noxious aliment, or vitiated secretion,
will have the effect of diminishing its muscular energy.
It is in this way that a draught of cold water, or a
quantity of ice, may at once paralyse the stomach. In
cases, therefore, of protracted indigestion, it is evident
that both the *chemical* and *mechanical* functions of the
stomach will be injured; neither the one nor the other
can long remain alone affected. Irritation of the nerves
will occasion vitiated secretion, and vitiated secretion will
become a source of irritation to the nerves.

264. We have seen the manner in which indigestion
may take place in the stomach; but there are cases in
which the secretions of that organ are perfectly performed,
and in which the muscular contractions of the stomach
are carried on with healthy vigour and regularity. The
chyme is, therefore, duly elaborated, and the paroxysm of
dyspepsia may not commence until the food has entered
the duodenum.

IMPERFECT DIGESTION IN THE DUODENUM.

265. In the earlier part of this work, the structure,
position, and functions of this " *second stomach,*" have
been fully described, and the practitioner must bear in
mind the peculiar circumstances which relate to its
anatomy and physiology, in order to understand the

nature and extent of those aberrations to which it is liable. The chyme certainly undergoes some change in this organ, independent of that which is produced on it by its admixture with the bile and pancreatic juice, and which would appear to be effected by the agency of its own peculiar secretion; this secretion may become insufficient in quantity to answer its intended purpose, or its quality may be occasionally vitiated; but there exists no direct evidence upon this point, and we can only maintain the probability of such an occurrence on the ground of analogy. As far as the pathology of this organ is concerned, I consider the contributions of Dr. Yeats, in his paper published in the Medical Transactions, as truly valuable; and I have great pleasure in bearing testimony of its importance. The hints which I have derived from it, have not only been useful to me, in the execution of my present task, but in the prosecution of my duties as a private practitioner. I am quite satisfied, that many morbid affections which have been usually attributed to the stomach, ought to be solely referred to the functional aberrations of the duodenum; and when we consider the situation of this intestine, with respect to the colon, and the pressure which it must suffer whenever this latter gut is loaded with fæces; when we reflect upon the elaborate manner in which it is constructed; the connexion of its nerves with other organs; its limited capacity and motion; its tortuous course; the distress which must arise from its distension, and the irritation which, from such a cause, must be immediately propagated through its nerves to very important parts; when we remember that the pancreatic and biliary ducts may be obstructed by its repletion, and the necessary flow of the bile prevented; and, lastly, when we consider that the *vena cava inferior* may be thus pressed upon, and the circulation of its blood obstructed, — we shall not have much hesitation in admitting that a morbid condition of the duodenum must prove a pregnant source of local as well as of general distress. It is also necessary to state that, from the confinement which this intestine suffers at its termination within the ring, at the mesentery, the propulsion of its contents is liable to be retarded or obstructed; and, should any hard or indigestible matter have escaped the action of the stomach, it may, by lodging, occasion a temporary stoppage in this part of the canal.

266. The symptoms, which arise from *duodenal* indigestion, are easily distinguishable from those which depend upon an affection of the stomach. In a casual paroxysm of this kind, the distress is not felt until some time has elapsed after the indigestible meal, and then no oppression is felt at the pit of the stomach, but on the right side, and a puffiness is frequently perceptible in the region occupied by the intestine. In some cases a severe pain is felt in the back, especially in the region of the right kidney; and Dr. Yeats states a symptom, which I have also noticed on such occasions—a faint and fluttering pulse, occasioned by the pressure of the *vena cava* against the spine by the distended intestine. Emetics in such a case are safer remedies than purgatives; by their action, the offending substance is regurgitated into the stomach, and thus at once eliminated; whereas a purgative may increase the distress, and even produce farther mischief. Glysters, however, will be always advisable, in order to remove any pressure which the colon may occasion by its indurated contents.

267. I believe that where indigestion in the stomach has remained for any considerable length of time, that the duodenum rarely escapes corresponding mischief; it is difficult to imagine a case in which the fluids of the stomach are constantly in a vitiated, and those of the duodenum in a healthy condition. The very circumstance of half-concocted chyme being repeatedly urged forward into the cavity of the intestine, will be sufficient to de-

range its functions. When, therefore, we take a general view of the symptoms which mark confirmed digestion, we must take into consideration the effects produced by the derangement of this important organ. In some cases the evidence of such an affection will be more striking than in others, but in most we shall find some proof of its existence.

268. A casual indigestion in the duodenum may be produced by various causes; in addition to those already enumerated as capable of occasioning such an affection in the stomach, we may mention mechanical obstruction, arising from the presence of nuts, cherry-stones, &c.; a vitiated state of the bile, or a temporary suspension of its flow from the liver, by which the chyme will be prevented from undergoing its destined changes, and thus, remaining in the duodenum, may ferment, and distend the intestine with air; accumulations also in the colon, which, by diminishing the diameter of the duodenum, will necessarily impede its functions.

OF HEADACHS WHICH ARISE FROM INDIGESTION.

269. From the intimate sympathy which subsists between the nerves of the stomach and the brain, it is not extraordinary that any casual derangement of the digestive process should communicate its influence to the head. Dr. Warren * has described this complaint with an accuracy which, as far as description goes, leaves nothing to be desired. He states that there are two forms of dyspeptic headach; the one he refers to a fault in the stomach, the other to a defective action of the upper bowels. The former is distinguished by a languid and feeble, but not an unnaturally frequent pulse; the tongue is whitish and slightly coated; the edges are of a pale red colour. The

* Medical Transactions, vol. iv. p. 233.

patient perceives a sensation of mistiness before the eyes, and general indistinctness of vision; he feels a dull pain or weight in the head, attended with some confusion, is slightly giddy, and fearful of falling. These symptoms are attended with slight nausea, or an uneasiness and sense of irritation in the stomach; and often also by a feeling of constriction about the fauces, accompanied with a watery secretion from the posterior part of the mouth. Coldness, slight stiffness or numbness of the fingers, are sometimes present; and the other parts of the system are, in general, affected with a great degree of nervous sensibility. The second species of headach, or that depending upon irritation in the bowels, probably in the duodenum, is remarkable for the appearance of brilliant ocular spectra which distress the patient; there is chilliness of the body, and coldness and dampness of the hands and feet; the pain in the head is very severe, attended with a sensation of coldness and tightness of the scalp, slight giddiness, weight, distension and stiffness of the eye-balls. In some cases, as these symptoms increase, they are accompanied by tingling and numbness of the fingers and hand. The tongue, in this disorder, is usually covered with a yellow-ish white fur, and is often very considerably coated with it. The pulse is of the natural frequency, but languid; nausea is often present, but seldom in so great a degree as to produce vomiting. There is usually flatulency, and a sensation of dryness and inactivity of the bowels. This last symptom I consider as pathognomonic; the patient feels as if his bowels had lost their sensibility, and were unable to propel their contents, which occasions a peculiar sensation of weight and stoppage. Dr. Warren observes, that the appearances of the stools vary so much, that a general rule cannot be drawn from them; but he believes, that in all cases of headach of this description, they will be found of an unhealthy quality. The most frequent appearance in them is bile in too large quantity; some-

times of various colours, and of different degrees of viscidity; occasionally the evacuations have a natural appearance, but contain portions of undigested food. At other
times, the stools are of a faint yellow colour, and float
upon water, giving out an odour like that of saliva: a
very common appearance, especially where there has been
great dejection of spirits, is a loose stool, of a dark green-
ish-brown colour, in smell resembling that of the grounds
of sour beer.

270. The *stomach* headach generally occurs in the
earlier stage of digestion; that which may be termed the
duodenal headach, takes place when the food has passed
into the intestine. The former is relieved by an emetic,
the latter receives no mitigation from such a remedy; this
is consonant with our theory of its origin; whereas, a
purgative, as we should expect, generally cuts short the
paroxysm, by hastening the expulsion of the offending
cause.

271. From the symptoms above related, the practitioner will not be at a loss to discriminate between these
two species of headach; but pain in the head may arise
from causes distinct from the alimentary canal; as from
congestion of the brain, from its internal disorganization,
from diseased bones of the skull, or from a deranged state
of the nervous system. It will be useful to point out the
diagnostic symptoms by which each of these affections
may be distinguished. Dr. Warren observes, that head-
achs which arise from congestion of the brain, are distinguished from those of dyspeptic origin, by the presence of
plethoric symptoms, by a full and oppressed pulse, by a
difference in the character of the pain, which, in the headach arising from fulness of blood, is accompanied with
throbbing, and a sense of action in the system, which
alarms the feelings; while the pain of dyspeptic head-
achs is described as being either a dull aching, or else a

racking pain, often moving from one part of the head to another, and attended with soreness of the scalp. In the first, the eyes look red and full; in the second, they have a depressed and languid appearance. Those which arise from internal disorganization, the same eminent physician considers to be marked by an acute fixed pain, by a quick, irritable, and sometimes irregular pulse ; but should pressure on the brain have taken place, the pulse is full and slow, but is not attended with the steady violent heat which accompanies sudden congestion of blood in that organ. When headach is caused by chronic disease of the bones of the skull, it is distinguished by the constancy of the pain, which is confined to one spot, whence violent shootings proceed to some fixed point. As the disorder advances, slight symptoms of pressure on the brain ensue; and on examination, a tenderness of the bone is observed. The nervous headach is distinguished by the absence of constitutional disorder, and by the smallness of the space on the surface of the head which the pain occupies.

272. There sometimes occurs a soreness of the scalp, with shooting pains, which are produced by the slightest touch. This affection, I believe, always depends upon some derangement of the biliary system.

273. There is a species of headach which would appear to depend upon a languid circulation through the brain; it occurs after an excess of wine; or, in women, during the catamenial discharge. It is described as rather resembling numbness than pain, or that sensation which is produced by intense cold. The languor of the circulation, pallor of the countenance, and other symptoms of debility, will offer sufficient means for distinguishing it.

274. If the dyspeptic headach be allowed to take its course, it will generally terminate in a few hours; but when it has become habitual, it is often protracted through one, two, or more days. Its cure is to be effected

by those means which we have afterwards to consider, as the best modes of rectifying the errors of the digestive organs.

275. Cutaneous eruptions are not unfrequently produced by a fit of indigestion ; such affections are popularly denominated *surfeits;* they are generally of short duration, and disappear on the removal of the offending cause; although severe and inveterate diseases of the skin are sometimes established, and continued by a chronic disease of the stomach or other digestive organs. The best mode of treating such affections, and the diet which should be employed for their cure, will form a subject for future consideration.

Indigestion from Biliary Derangement.

276. It is evident that a regular and healthy secretion of bile is indispensable to the act of chylification, and to the proper action of the intestines, and that a deficiency, redundancy, or a vitiated condition of this fluid, may act as an exciting cause of indigestion. If it be deficient, the chyme cannot undergo that decomposition in the duodenum by which chyle is formed and separated ; and as the bowels are, at the same time, deprived of their natural stimulus, the undigested mass is not protruded, but is left to undergo various morbid changes ; air is extricated, the alimentary secretions become depraved, and the whole series of the digestive functions are thus suspended, or deranged. If the bile be too copiously secreted, it is poured out in large quantities into the intestine, producing temporary diarrhœa, and part of it being regurgitated into the stomach, during the act of vomiting, which, in the first instance, is excited by the sympathy of the stomach with the duodenum and hepatic system, occasions a train of symptoms of greater or less severity, according to the circumstances of each particular case. If the bile be

vitiated in quality, it will not only be incapable of accomplishing the alimentary change which it is destined to fulfil, but it will irritate and fret the mucous membrane by its contact. It is evident that the violence and extent of the symptoms produced by such causes will be liable to vary; and the practitioner must not imagine, that the absence of diarrhœa, colic, and other violent feelings, affords evidence of the healthy state of the biliary secretions. Derangements in these functions often proceed insidiously, and lay the foundation for a serious disease, which, although latent for a period, will ultimately be kindled into activity, whenever an exciting cause shall fire the train.

277 To explain the origin of biliary irregularities, we have to consider the sympathies by which the liver may be influenced. The investigation of the diseases of warm climates, and the corrected views, with regard to the autumnal complaints of our climate, have sufficiently established the existence of a sympathy between the skin and the liver. Whenever an organ has been in a state of over-excitement, it is liable to fall into a corresponding state of torpor. The perspiration is, therefore, more apt to be checked after the continuance of hot weather, than at any other season of the year; and since the same observation may be extended to the liver, we shall readily perceive the cause of those biliary affections which so generally occur in this country during the autumnal season. The application of cold to the feet, or whatever contributes to check the perspiratory functions, may create, in those predisposed to such complaints, a *bilious* attack. The sympathy which subsists between the stomach and liver, has already been adverted to. It seems a wise provision, that the biliary function should be connected, by a close sympathy, with that of the stomach, in order that the food, converted into chyme, may meet with a necessary quantity of bile in the duodenum. In consequence of such a sympathy, irrita-

tion in the stomach is generally attended with an increased secretion of bile ; the action of nausea is usually
followed by such an effect. Hence, melted butter, every
thing fried, pastry, and other indigestible materials, are
popularly denominated *bilious;* and although such a term
countenances a latitude of expression, which is inconsistent with the more definite notions of strict pathology,
yet it cannot be said to be erroneous. As the varied and
increased action of a gland has much influence in deter-
mining the nature of the fluid secreted, we cannot be at a
loss to explain the vitiated condition in which the bile is
secreted under such circumstances; indeed, it is frequently on such occasions of a degenerated colour, extremely
acrid, and scarcely possessing the qualities of bile. Dr.
Saunders considers it probable, that from the quantity
secreted, and the rapid manner in which it is poured into
the duodenum, there is not time sufficient for a perfect
secretion.

278. We may therefore agree with Dr. Saunders, that
whenever, either from an irregular distribution of nervous
energy, or from the operation of indigestible and acescent
food, the tone of the stomach falls below the degree
necessary to the digestive process, the liver immediately
sympathises with it, and bile is no longer emulged into
the duodenum, until a reaction takes place, when its
quantity is morbidly increased in proportion to the degree
of previous atony. If this occur to such an extent, that
its free admission into the intestine be impeded, it will
accumulate in the excretory ducts of the liver, and either
regurgitate into the system by the hepatic veins, or be
absorbed by the lymphatic system, and a yellow suffusion
of the skin will follow.

279. The abuse of spirituous liquors, from their operation on the stomach and brain, is a fertile cause of
biliary derangement, and from the sympathy between
the sensorium and the liver, the effects of strong and

sudden mental emotions, in occasioning an irregular secretion of bile, will also admit of satisfactory explanation.

Progress and Symptoms of Chronic Indigestion.

280. From considering a fit of indigestion in the stomach or duodenum, let us now proceed to trace its consequences, when it is frequently repeated or protracted. In this case, other organs become successively involved in the mischief, and a train of distressing and complicated symptoms arise. Dr. Wilson Philip has considered indigestion as divisible into three distinct stages. Under the first, he arranges those symptoms which merely announce a disturbed and unhealthy condition of the digestive functions. The second stage he considers as denoted by the tenderness of the epigastrium, and the hardness of the pulse. The third stage includes those diseases which he supposes to arise from the change of structure, which is ultimately produced by long-continued functional derangement. I have no great objection to a conventional division of this kind, if it can in any way assist the memory of the practitioner, and contribute to the perspicuity of the description, by presenting the symptoms in well-defined groups, rather than in a separate and unconnected form. But the arrangement is wholly artificial. Nature does not acknowledge it, nor will she submit to it; if, then, any advantage is to be derived from it, it must be received and considered only as an attempt to class together those symptoms which may arise from functional aberration, and those which are more usually associated with organic change. We must renounce all rigid adherence to definite stages, and arbitrary divisions, which nature disclaims. Every practitioner of any experience must well know that the hard pulse and tenderness of the epigastrium are likely to occur in even a temporary attack

of indigestion; and I have frequently witnessed extensive mischief, with change of structure, without the occurrence of such indications. With regard to the " third stage," I would observe, that if the diseases therein stated as the results of indigestion, be purely such, we may as well, at once, refer all organic disease to the same source, and, like the ancient physicians of Egypt, confine our prescriptions to vomits, purgatives, and abstinence. I am well aware how unpopular must be any doctrine that opposes such a belief, for I have practised too much in the western part of Cornwall, not to know the consolation which phthisical patients derive from being assured that their complaints owe their origin to a disordered stomach ; but although the physician may reconcile his conscience thus piously to deceive his patient, let him be aware how he deceives himself. I make these observations in the pure spirit of philosophic candour; I respect and duly appreciate the talents of Dr. Philip; I give him every possible credit for the good intention and integrity with which he advances his opinions, and I feel well assured that he will extend the same charity to me; but I differ with him. Indigestion, or, in other words, derangement of the stomach, is a frequent companion of pulmonary disease, and what is the disease in which the stomach does not sympathise? but I am sceptical as to the existence of any malady which is entitled to the specific appellation of " *dyspeptic phthisis.*" A person having tubercles in the lungs may have his life protracted for many years, by judicious management, and by avoiding every exciting cause which might kindle the spark into flame, by keeping the circulation in check, and promoting the healthy action of the secretions. On the contrary, the fatal termination may be equally accelerated by want of care, and, above all, by creating a permanent disturbance in the digestive functions. If Dr. Philip designates a latent disease, thus kindled into activity, " *dyspeptic phthisis,*" I have no objec-

tion to the term ; we are no longer at issue, our difference
of opinion is not essential; it is an affair of words, and of
words only.   But to return from this digression to the
subject more immediately before us, viz. the complicated
train of symptoms which successively present themselves
in cases of protracted dyspepsia.

281. It has been seen that indigestion may originate
in the stomach, or intestines, either from vitiated secretion,
muscular imbecility, nervous derangement, or biliary and
pancreatic disturbance; but, from whatever cause the
disease may primarily originate, after it has remained for
some time in operation, the different organs, directly or
sympathetically connected with the chylopoietic apparatus,
will participate in the mischief, and it will not be easy
to distinguish between primary symptoms, and those of
mere induction.   There is, perhaps, not any disease which
is more protiform in its aspects than dyspepsia : we shall
rarely find any two cases precisely similar in the origin
and progress of their symptoms, although to an experienced
judge they will present such a general similitude, as to
leave no doubt of their nature and causes.

282. The dyspeptic patient having, for some time,
suffered from those feelings of uneasiness, which have
been already described (254), experiences some diminution
in his strength.   This, at first, is only occasional, and is
for awhile attributed by him to some accidental circumstance ;   he had felt it before, and the readiness with
which his elasticity and strength returned, naturally in-
spires a hope that his present depression may be removed ;
but it has endured longer than usual, and he ultimately
becomes alarmed.   It is in this stage of the malady, that
the patient frequently introduces himself, for the first
time, to a physician.   It is of great importance, upon such
an occasion, to distinguish between that feeling of transient
depression, which as Tissot observes, is invariably associated with alimentary disturbance, and that debility which

announces a general diminution of constitutional energy.
In the former case, there are periods in which the patient
feels perfectly well and strong; but in the latter, although
his spirits may vary, he never rises to the healthy standard
of vigour. He tells you, that " he begins to feel his usual
avocations irksome, and too laborious; that he has long
suffered from a *bad digestion,*" which by care and
management he had been hitherto enabled to control; but
that he has now little or no appetite, that his strength
fails him, and that he fears he is " getting into a bad way."
He finds that the slightest exercise occasions fatigue, and
deluges him with perspiration. On examining the tongue,
it will be usually found coated on the posterior part, and
on its centre, with a brownish-yellow fur; his bowels are,
by turns, costive, and too much relaxed; the pulse at this
period is generally slow and small; although it is sometimes hard; his countenance is more pallid than usual;
the eyes appear sunken, and the eye-lids swollen, and the
eye-balls are occasionally injected with yellow streaks.

In some cases, heartburn and a sense of oppression are
experienced after meals; but in others, the patient only
complains of languor and extreme listlessness. On some
occasions, a sense of constriction is felt about the fauces,
and a difficulty of swallowing is experienced, as if the
œsophagus presented some mechanical obstruction to the
passage of food. Dizziness; unusual drowsiness; pains
in the head; ringing in the ears; a disagreeable taste in
the mouth; an altered state of the salivary secretion, being
sometimes limpid like water, and at others thick and
ropy; palpitation and a sense of faintness are symptoms
which, also, in a greater or less degree, usually distress the
dyspeptic sufferer. His hands are alternately hot and
cold; in the former state they are dry, in the latter more
usually damp. His nights are sometimes, but not generally,
disturbed by restlessness and uneasy dreams. He wakes
in the morning without that feeling of refreshment which

follows repose in health, and is unwilling to rise from his
bed, or indeed to move; his limbs ache, the muscles of
the trunk are even sore to the touch; and any change of
position is attended with inconvenience.   Every alteration
in the weather is felt as a serious evil; if it becomes a
degree or two colder, he creeps to the fire, and inveighs,
in terms of bitterness and sarcasm, against the variable-
ness of the climate; if its temperature be raised, he is
oppressed with heat.   His bowels become more and more
untractable;   the usual purgative ceases to produce its
accustomed effect; he increases the dose, and when it does
operate, the action is too powerful, and its effects are not
easily checked; a diarrhœa is established; and this again,
in its turn, is superseded by still more obstinate constipation.   If I could but obtain a medicine, cries the invalid
to his physician, that would keep my bowels in a regular
state, I should soon become convalescent: there lies the
difficulty; the evil arises from the inconstant and unsettled
state of the alimentary secretions, and it is not easy to
graduate an artificial stimulant so that it shall always
correspond with the varying state of the organs upon
which it is to operate.   The depression of his spirits
increases as the disease advances; he gives his case up as
lost; loses flesh, suffers a thousand distressing sensations,
and fancies the existence of a thousand more.   Wandering
pains are felt in the bowels and side; a tenderness in the
epigastrium is experienced on pressure; the abdomen is
often preternaturally tense; his breathing is occasionally
oppressed; a short dry cough distresses him, and expecto-
ration is extremely difficult. If, under such circumstances,
the alvine discharges be inspected, they may present every
variety of morbid appearance; they may be unnatural in
colour, odour, consistence, figure, or quantity.   I shall,
hereafter, have occasion to speak more fully upon this
subject, as well as upon the morbid appearances which
the urine presents under such circumstances.

283. The patient, in this stage of his complaint, will sometimes complain of being disturbed, on first falling asleep,
by fearful startings, and catching of the limbs, uneasiness
in the region of the chest, attended with difficulty of
breathing, so as to resemble *angina pectoris;* and it is not
unusual for him on such occasions to perceive flashes of
fire, like lightning, with a numbness in his hands ; this
numbness is sometimes only felt in one or two fingers.
Sore throat, occasioned by relaxation, is also a very usual
symptom ; the skin is frequently dry, and even scaly ; the
tongue also becomes drier, and sometimes clean, and of a
brighter colour than usual. Harrassed by such feelings,
the unhappy invalid anxiously proposes a trial of change
of air, and his friends acquiesce in the belief that such a
plan will tend to his recovery. He quits his residence, but
to no purpose, his emaciation increases ; his ancles swell ;
and the general debility thus produced sooner or later
calls some other disease into activity, the nature and
locality of which will necessarily vary in different cases.
If the spring of a piece of machinery snaps, and all its
different parts are hurried into violent motion, the wheel
upon which the greatest strain is made, or that which is of
the weakest construction, will be the first to give way:
Just so is it with the human body. Those organs more
immediately connected with the digestive function will
more readily undergo a change of structure, on account of
the protracted irritation they must have sustained. Then,
in succession, those which are connected by the ties of
sympathy ; while the general loss of balance, thus occasioned, will render any organ, originally weak, very liable
to disease. This view of the subject is supported by experience ; the history of those complaints which terminate
the life of the dyspeptic patient, will sufficiently explain
the manner in which they were produced. Unless they
take their origin in a viscus immediately connected with

the digestive functions, as in the stomach, intestines, mesenteric glands, liver, &c. dyspepsia can only be considered in the light of a general debilitating cause; and it is a circumstance no less extraordinary than important, that when *any new disease is permanently established, the original symptoms are mitigated, and sometimes wholly suspended; whereas, if the new affection be only symptomatic, instead of relieving, it often aggravates them.*

284. Dr. Philip lays great stress upon the hardness of the pulse, as indicative of approaching mischief; I confess that my experience does not confirm the importance he has ascribed to it. The permanent tenderness of the epigastrium, and a clean bright tongue, always excite a greater apprehension in my mind. The pulse is very treacherous in its indications : I have found it to be soft and undulating in cases where no doubt could exist as to the presence of organic mischief. It is just, however, to state that Dr. Philip acknowledges that its hardness is sometimes only perceptible when examined in a particular way. He says that those who have been much in the habit of examining the different states of the pulse, must be aware, that its hardness is most perceptible when a slight degree of pressure is employed. A certain degree, by greatly compressing the vessel, will give some feeling of softness to the hardest pulse, and a slight degree of hardness is not perceptible with the pressure generally employed in feeling the pulse. If the pressure be gradually lessened till it comes to nothing, it often happens that a hardness of pulse is felt before the pulse wholly vanishes under the finger, when no hardness can be perceived in the usual way of feeling it.

285. I consider the train of reasoning by which Dr. Philip establishes the important fact, that *long-continued irritation at length terminates in inflammation and organic derangement in the part affected,*—as constituting a very

valuable part of his work. The idea is certainly not new, but the cases which he has adduced in illustration of its truth, are apposite and very satisfactory. The practical mischief which arises from a neglect of the fact is, I am satisfied, very extensive.

286. After indigestion has continued to harrass the stomach for some time, its villous coat becomes affected, and as the pylorus, from the peculiar nature of its office, is more exposed to the continued source of irritation than other parts of the stomach, it is certainly, as Dr. Philip justly states, very liable to become inflamed, and the tenderness in the epigastrium may perhaps in some cases be thus explained; but it must be remembered that, in internal diseases, the pain is frequently referred to a part at some distance from the real source of it; a morbid distention of the liver, an irritated state of duodenum, and a gorged condition of the colon, are not uncommonly attended with the same feeling. It is, at the same time, difficult to imagine, how serious mischief can be inflicted upon the pylorus without the occurrence of vomiting.

287. When the bowels have been long in a state of disorder, the villous coat becomes tumid, turgid with blood, and sometimes ulcerated; and Mr. Abernethy states that these appearances have been most manifest in the large intestines. He says that he has repeatedly observed, in dissections of these cases, the large intestines to be more diseased than the smaller ones, and he accounts for this fact in the following manner. If digestion is incomplete, the indigested food must be liable to chemical changes, and the products resulting from this cause are likely to be most stimulating to the large intestines. Indeed, he adds, in advanced stages of this disorder, mucus and jelly tinged with blood are discharged, and it seems probable that a kind of chronic dysentery may be thus induced. In my own practice, I have witnessed several cases of this kind; but I confess that I cannot perceive

why the duodenum and smaller intestines should not be equally exposed to such a source of irritation.

288. It is not extraordinary that protracted dyspepsia should sometimes terminate in a disease of the mesenteric glands; it is only surprising that such a state of irritation and imperfect development of chyle should continue for so long a period, as they are in many cases known to do, without occasioning such an effect. We must suppose that the selecting tact with which the lacteals are endowed, enables them for a considerable time to reject imperfectly formed or vitiated chyle, and that it is not until this is destroyed, that the irritating matter finds its way to the glands. The circulating fluids of the body are for the same reason not materially deteriorated until the dyspeptic disease has continued for some time; the blood then undergoes some important change, but animal chemistry is not yet sufficiently advanced to demonstrate its nature. I have examined the blood of a patient who had long laboured under a disease of the digestive organs, and the most remarkable character which it presented was the loose texture of its crassamentum, and a deficiency in its red globules. In some cases the serum assumes an opaline appearance.

289. When we consider the connection which subsists between the function of the kidneys and that of the chylopoietic organs, we shall easily explain the disturbed appearance of the urine, and the occurrence of calculous disorders in cases of dyspepsia.

290. Before I proceed to consider the medical treatment and dietetic regulations most appropriate for the cure of the several forms of indigestion, it will be necessary to inquire into the remote and immediate causes of that disease. In fulfilling this part of my duty, I shall deviate from the usual plan of such investigations, and arrange my observations in an order that may, in some degree, correspond with that which should be adopted by

every physician who undertakes to examine a patient with a view to detect the cause, nature, and seat of his disease. I shall first present the reader with a tabular arrangement of the objects of such an inquiry, and then comment upon the relative importance of each.

A SCHEME

FOR INVESTIGATING THE CAUSES, NATURE, AND SEAT
OF INDIGESTION.

I. LEADING QUESTIONS, *concerning*

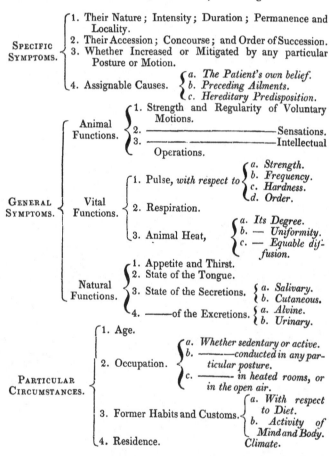

SPECIFIC SYMPTOMS.

1. Their Nature; Intensity; Duration; Permanence and Locality.
2. Their Accession; Concourse; and Order of Succession.
3. Whether Increased or Mitigated by any particular Posture or Motion.
4. Assignable Causes.
 - a. *The Patient's own belief.*
 - b. *Preceding Ailments.*
 - c. *Hereditary Predisposition.*

GENERAL SYMPTOMS.

Animal Functions.
1. Strength and Regularity of Voluntary Motions.
2. ————————————Sensations.
3. ———— ————————Intellectual Operations.

Vital Functions.
1. Pulse, *with respect to*
 - a. *Strength.*
 - b. *Frequency.*
 - c. *Hardness.*
 - d. *Order.*
2. Respiration.
3. Animal Heat,
 - a. *Its Degree.*
 - b. *— Uniformity.*
 - c. *— Equable dif- fusion.*

Natural Functions.
1. Appetite and Thirst.
2. State of the Tongue.
3. State of the Secretions.
 - a. *Salivary.*
 - b. *Cutaneous.*
4. ————of the Excretions.
 - a. *Alvine.*
 - b. *Urinary.*

PARTICULAR CIRCUMSTANCES.

1. Age.
2. Occupation.
 - a. *Whether sedentary or active.*
 - b. *————conducted in any particular posture.*
 - c. *———— in heated rooms, or in the open air.*
3. Former Habits and Customs.
 - a. *With respect to Diet.*
 - b. *Activity of Mind and Body.*
4. Residence. Climate.

II. OCCASIONAL QUESTIONS, *concerning*

FEMALES.
1. State of Menstrual Discharge.
2. Married or Unmarried State.
3. Impregnation. Lactation. Number of Children.

CHILDREN. 1. Dentition. 2. Former Diseases. 3. Diet, &c.

III. GENERAL OBSERVATIONS, *upon*

Physical
Character. { 1. Bulk and Stature. 2. Particular Conformation.
3. Complexion and Physiognomy. 4. Mobility and
Irritability.

IV. COLLATERAL CIRCUMSTANCES.

1. Season of the Year. 2. Nature of Prevailing Epidemics.

3. Weather. { *a. Moisture and Dryness.*
b. Prevailing Winds.
c. Abundance and quality of Fruits.

A COMMENTARY UPON THE PRECEDING TABLE.

291. In order to illustrate the relative importance of
the several subjects which are embraced in the preceding
tabular scheme, as well as to direct the practitioner into
the more direct path of pathological inquiry, let us suppose
a person, labouring under some one of the forms of dyspepsia, to present himself for examination. We first learn,
from his own report, the general nature of the symptoms
by which he is distressed; and we then proceed to make
such farther inquiries as may enable us to form an opinion
respecting their origin and mode of cure.

292. The *intensity* of the symptoms cannot be always
inferred from the patient's own report, but must be deduced from our experience in such cases. The dyspeptic is too apt to depict his feelings in extravagant
language, and to become unnecessarily anxious and ap-
prehensive. An inquiry into the *duration* of his complaints is of much importance; for it has been already
stated (283) that the intervals of comfort are abridged as
the disease progresses, until at length he becomes harrassed by an uninterrupted series of sufferings. It is,
however, from the *locality* of the symptoms that we are to
form our opinion with respect to their seat and origin;
and for ascertaining this fact we must be particular in our
inquiry, and minute in our examination. Is the stomach
affected? If a sense of weight or burning after the inges-

tion of food, acid, or putrescent eructations be present, we may conclude such to be the case. If there exist any uneasiness or fulness in the epigastric and right hypochondric regions, produced or increased by pressure, we may infer that there exists some diseased condition of the liver, duodenum, or, perhaps, of the pyloric orifice of the stomach; and that we may be enabled, under such circumstances, to form a diagnosis, the patient must be submitted to a manual examination. For this purpose, every ligature must be removed from the abdomen, and he must be placed on a sofa, reclining on his back, with his legs drawn up, so as to throw the abdominal muscles into a state of relaxation. Where the fulness and tenderness arise from a distended state of duodenum, the sensation given to the hand is very different from that which is produced by organic disease of the liver; the tumor in the former case is more diffused and less defined. Dr. Yeats also justly observes, that, by pressure *on* the region of the liver, no uneasiness will be complained of, but if the pressure be made with the edge of the open hand under the ribs, with the palm of it flat upon the abdomen, considerable uneasiness will be felt up towards the liver, and down towards the right kidney; a soreness is likewise felt an inch or two to the right, just above the navel. In such cases also, the anatomical accuracy with which the patient will trace the course of the duodenum with his finger, from the stomach to the loins on the right side, and back again across the abdomen to the umbilicus, will greatly assist the diagnosis. There are, besides, other symptoms to be hereafter enumerated which will enable us to arrive at a still more positive conclusion. It is of the greatest importance to distinguish between a morbid state of the duodenum and that of the liver: I have frequently, in the course of my own practice, seen patients who have undergone salivation, from a belief in the existence of hepatic disease, but who were merely suffering under duodenal irritation; and my friend Dr. Yeats has stated the same conviction upon the subject. On the other hand, I am equally satisfied that chronic inflammation of the liver has been repeatedly mistaken for a dyspeptic state of the stomach. Dr. Saunders says, that he has seen many cases of this kind, which have been supposed to arise from indigestion. The patient generally complains of pain, which he falsely attributes to the stomach; and its continuance is so short, and the degree of it frequently so inconsiderable, that no alarm respecting the future health of the patient is produced. The relief obtained by eructation and discharge of air, tends to confirm the opinion that the seat of the disease is in the stomach; but this relief may be explained on the principle of removing the distention of the stomach, and so taking off the pressure of this organ from that which is the seat of the complaint.

293. Where the tenderness in the epigastrium is extremely circumscribed, not occupying a space larger than a shilling, Dr. Philip infers the presence of an inflammatory affection, or a state approaching to it, of the pylorus, excited by the passage of the irritating contents of the stomach. I have already expressed some doubt upon this subject; I cannot conceive such a state of pylorus, as to occasion pain on pressure, to be unattended with vomiting.

294. *The accession, concourse, and order of succession* of the different symptoms, are calculated to throw considerable light upon the nature of a dyspeptic disease; indeed, in protracted cases, it is only by a careful examination of these circumstances that we shall be able to separate primary from secondary affections. The stomach cannot long err without communicating its vice to the other chylopoietic organs; the liver may become affected from mere irritation, and every part of the body, from sympathetic influence, may put on the appearance of disease. How are we then, except by a careful examina-

tion into the history of the case, to ascertain the organ in which the mischief originated?

295. *Whether the symptoms are mitigated, or increased by any particular posture or motion.* This is an important question. Where the disease is confined to the stomach, the patient appears capable of lying with equal ease on either side : but if the duodenum or liver be affected, he will experience some uneasiness on lying on the left side. Where the disease has become complicated, lying on either side is irksome, and the easiest position is found to be that of lying on the back, with the shoulders a little raised, and inclined to the right side. The muscles of the chest are, on such occasions, not unfrequently sore, and the patient finds it difficult to turn even in his bed without pain.

296. *Assignable causes.* It will be always right to inquire of the patient whether he can account for the accession of his disease. He will tell you whether he has exposed himself to the operation of any of those causes which are known to be active in producing it. His previous state of health should also be investigated, for we may be thus enabled to explain the occurrence of symptoms, and to connect them with the derangements of distant organs. An affection of the stomach may, for instance, be traced to some sympathetic action, which might otherwise be mistaken for a primary disease.

297. *Hereditary susceptibility.* So many vague notions are entertained upon this subject, that it will be necessary for me to define the latitude in which the term is to be received. Dyspepsia, depending upon peculiarity of stomach, is certainly hereditary, but it is only hereditary in *predisposition*, always requiring the influence of some cause to produce it, and consequently always to be prevented, and often relieved, by avoiding the exciting cause. In cases of great obscurity, a knowledge of the disease to which the patient's parent is particularly ob-

noxious, must, for reasons sufficiently obvious, assist our judgment.

298. Having acquired all the information which is to be obtained by questioning the patient upon the subject of his " specific symptoms," we are next to investigate the " general symptoms," connected with the animal, vital, and natural functions. In this line of inquiry, the judgment which we have been able to form will be confirmed or modified; we shall, at the same time, be enabled to discover the influence which the local affection has produced upon the general system.

299. It has been already observed (283) that the strength of the patient, both as it regards the voluntary motions, and intellectual operations, does not suffer until the dyspeptic disease has acquired a considerable influence over the system. The condition, therefore, of these functions will serve as a measure of the severity of the complaint; but in forming such an estimate we must be careful to avoid the fallacies with which it is surrounded (283).

300. *The pulse* only affords indications of questionable value; when taken in conjunction with other symptoms it may serve to fortify our conclusions; but I am anxious to impress my strong conviction upon the mind of the practitioner, that when received as an isolated testimony, it will be liable to lead him into error. Its strength, when other evidences concur, will undoubtedly throw some light upon the general state of the vital powers ; its frequency may indicate a state of morbid excitement, its *hardness* must excite the suspicion of organic mischief, and its irregularity will denote a disturbed state of the circulation, the cause of which must be deduced from other symptoms.

301. *The state of the respiration* is a circumstance worthy of attention ; for it may concur, with other symptoms, to indicate a state of congestion in the abdominal viscera, by which the descent of the diaphragm is impeded. It will also suggest other states of primary or

secondary disease, the nature of which the reader will easily understand from the various observations which are interspersed through the preceding pages of this work.

302. *Animal heat.* The degree, uniformity, and equable diffusion of heat are circumstances of some importance : they will enable us to form some estimate of the state of the vital powers generally ; and when we consider what an intimate connection subsists between the temperature of the body and the different stages of digestion, it will throw some light upon the comparative energy with which they are performed.

303. With regard to the indications afforded by the state of the appetite for solids or liquids, I have already delivered my opinions.

304. *The appearance of the tongue* has also been noticed in the preceding pages of this work ; it is natural to expect that a part, which is so immediately connected with the functions of the stomach, should be the first to exhibit a deranged condition in dyspepsia, and we accordingly find this to be the case. Baglivi has said that the pulse may deceive you, but that the indication afforded by the tongue is infallible. It greatly varies, however, in appearance, in different cases, and in different stages of the same case. When white and milky, it announces general irritation. When brown or dark coloured, foul congestions in the primæ viæ, or the presence of vitiated secretion ; and when unusually bright and shining, a morbid condition of the villous coat of the stomach or intestines, which is usually associated with, or is the precursor of, organic mischief ; for it indicates the presence of a degree of fever not commonly excited by the simple functional aberrations of the digestive organs. · In some cases the tongue is comparatively clean, but its cuticle loses its natural hue and transparency, and presents a sodden appearance : this generally depends upon the secretions having been for a considerable length of time in an unnatural state.

305. *The salivary secretion* is susceptible of various morbid conditions, to which the labours of the animal-chemist have not hitherto been directed (24); it is sometimes unnaturally ropy or viscid, so as to occasion an incessant hawking; at other times it is so preternaturally thin and copious, as to be discharged from the mouth in considerable quantities. I have lately seen a dyspeptic patient who declares, that his pillow is thoroughly wet in the morning with the discharge which takes place during the night: and yet dryness of the mouth, and a parched tongue, are amongst the most disagreeable of his symptoms, as if the secretion had lost the power of lubricating the parts to which it is applied. Frank states that he has known the saliva, when secreted in unnatural quantities, to have become saccharine.

306. *The state of the cutaneous discharge* is a circumstance of more importance than physicians usually assign to it. The reciprocal connexion which subsists between the functions of the skin and stomach is so obvious, that if the latter be deranged, the former is immediately affected, and vice versâ. It is the change produced upon the skin which assists in bestowing that peculiar physiognomy so characteristic of protracted indigestion; and amongst the most useful remedies in this disease, will be found those which are calculated to restore the healthy action of the cutaneous organs. When we remember that a person in health who takes eight pounds of aliment during the twenty-four hours, will discharge five of them by perspiration, we shall readily perceive how greatly the suspension or derangement of such a function must burthen the digestive organs.

307. *The condition of the excretions,* as to quantity and quality, is another object of important inquiry. I shall first describe the different appearances which the fæces may present in the various states of chylopoietic disturbance. On some occasions they will contain an

excessive quantity of bile, on others they will not be
sufficiently tinged with that secretion, and will therefore
assume a light yellow, or a clay-brown colour. They will
sometimes more particularly indicate by their appearance
the presence of vitiated secretion, and have a dark olive,
or a blackish-brown hue. In some cases they have so far
degenerated as to resemble pitch. Where the biliary secretion has been irregularly supplied, the fæces may
assume a partially coloured appearance. It is not unusual to notice mucous and gelatinous matter, accompanying, but not mixed with the fæces, and which have been
sometimes mistaken for worms. It must have derived its
origin from the alimentary membranes, or from the glands
situated in the canal. There is a very peculiar morbid
evacuation which I have occasionally witnessed, and
which has been described as resembling yeast in colour
and consistence. This frequently comes on suddenly, and
as suddenly departs; it is generally very profuse in quantity, and is usually preceded by uneasy sensations in the
alimentary canal. It would appear to be a morbid secretion of the intestinal juices during a torpid state of the
liver: although in one case in which I witnessed its occurrence, it was evidently connected with a diseased state
of the pancreas. I may, in this place, take notice of the
appearance of fat-like lumps of matter which are sometimes passed from the intestines. I suspect that they are
inspissated portions of mucus from the cœcum; I have, at
least, observed such evacuations to be accompanied by
pain in that region. In most cases of dyspepsia, the
stools will contain portions of undigested food, shewing at
once the failure of the assimilating powers. The odour of
the discharge is a circumstance of importance; a fœtid
stool indicates less permanent or extensive change, than
one which is deficient in the characteristic odour, and
yields a faint smell. The consistence of the fæces will
likewise be found to afford some useful signs. It has

been generally supposed that their dryness affords a proof that the nutritive part of the aliment has been duly absorbed : and there can be no doubt that such motions, if their colour be natural, should be considered as favourable in cases of indigestion. Boerhäave has remarked, that " people who complain of going too seldom to stool, and of voiding hard and dry fæces, complain without reason, because this proves the strength of their constitution." The least favourable consistence is that of a soft pudding, especially if the discharge of the motion be unattended with a feeling of relief corresponding with the quantity evacuated ; a sensation of something being retained, accompanied with that of a bearing down in the lower portions of the intestines, is not unusual upon such occasions. There is a peculiar appearance connected with this species of evacuation, which, I believe, has never been described in any work, nor indeed is it easy to convey by words its exact nature. It was first pointed out to me by Dr. Baillie, and I have since noticed it in numerous instances, and become satisfied of its immediate connexion with diseased secretion. The consistence of the motion is that of a pudding, but it is of unequal density in its different parts, and exhibits a surface as if it had been rasped by a file. I have still another form of fæces to describe, which would seem to depend upon a contraction of the intestine ; the excrement is hard, but having a diameter not much exceeding that of a tobacco-pipe. In protracted cases of dyspepsia, the occurrence of this appearance has given origin to a belief in the existence of stricture in the rectum : but I believe its cause is always seated in the higher portions of the large intestines. Some of my readers may perhaps consider the observations which I have been induced to offer upon the appearances of the feculent discharge as unnecessarily minute : but I am anxious to urge upon every practitioner the absolute necessity of such inspections. No one can successfully conduct the treatment of a severe dyspeptic complaint unless he submits to the performance of such a duty. All the great physicians of antiquity relied upon such a source of information for their guidance. Hippocrates carried the practice to such an extent as to have acquired from some of the wits of his age the appellation of σχατοφαγος, as Aristophanes had before named Esculapius. Some modern practitioners have, from the same scrupulous attention, been obnoxious to a similar charge; but I trust that no physician will be induced to swerve from the performance of a paramount duty by such intimidation.*

308. *The examination of the urine* is also a matter of considerable importance. Its appearance will not only assist us in forming a judgment respecting the seat of the dyspeptic disease; but, if carefully watched from day to day, will point out the beneficial changes which our plan of diet and medicine may have produced. It will also instruct us in the species of food which best agrees with the patient; for slight errors of diet, although imperceptible in other respects, are generally announced by obvious changes in the urinary deposits.

309. Without entering, with chemical minuteness, into the history of the changes which the urine undergoes under different conditions of the body, there are certain phenomena with which every practitioner ought to be well acquainted : these I shall briefly enumerate, and endeavour to point out the indications which they severally afford. The quantity evacuated during a given interval is the first question which presents itself; a diminished flow of deep coloured urine is invariably associated with febrile

---

* A atient may be so circumstanced, that the preservation of the fæces, for inspection, is attended with inconvenience. It is, therefore, worthy of notice, that a table-spoonful of sweet oil poured over them, by investing the surface with a film, effectually prevents evaporation, and the consequent stench they might otherwise occasion. This precaution should always be adopted in the wards of hospitals.

action; while an increased quantity of pale urine more generally indicates a peculiar state of nervous irritability, unattended with fever. In estimating, however, this circumstance, the practitioner will see the importance of inquiring into the vicarious excretion of the skin. Much has been written upon the subject of *albuminous* urine, or that in which a coagulum is produced by the application of heat; Dr. Blackall has maintained that it is connected with too great an action in some part of the system, and he considers that its occurrence in dropsy should be received as an indication of the necessity of blood-letting. I have met with several cases of dyspepsia, in which such a state of urine occurred, and I am disposed to believe with Dr. Prout that it is derived from the chyle. I have, at this time, two patients under my care, who have long suffered from the effects of tuberculated lungs; and during the progress of the present work, I examined their urine, and found in both cases that it was albuminous. We have, probably, too few data to lead us to a safe conclusion with regard to the cause of the phenomenon: but I am, at present, impressed with a belief that it arises from imperfect sanguification; the chyle not undergoing the necessary changes to convert it into perfect blood, is eliminated by the kidneys. It is essential in every case of protracted dyspepsia, to inquire into the state of the urinary secretion, in order to ascertain whether the patient may not be labouring under diabetes. So many valuable works have appeared upon this subject, that I consider it unnecessary to enter upon its history: but I should not discharge my duty to the professional reader, were I to omit noticing the concise but luminous chapter with which Dr. Prout has favoured us in his truly valuable work on the diseases of the urine.

310. But of all the changes of which the urine is susceptible, none perhaps are less equivocal, or more indicative of a deranged state of the alimentary functions,

than the deposit of lithic acid, either in an amorphous or crystalline form. Dr. Prout states that this acid, when in the former condition, is always in some state of combination, generally with ammonia; but when in the latter, it is nearly pure. He observes, that in healthy urine the lithic salt exists in such a proportion, as to be held in permanent solution at all ordinary temperatures; but that from particular causes affecting the health, its quantity is preternaturally increased, and the *excess* is deposited as the urine cools. Dr. Philip is inclined to account for its appearance in the urine from an increased quantity of acid passing through the urinary organs: from this view of the subject the lithic acid deposited must be considered as arising, not from the excess of that substance in the urine, but from a decomposition of the compounds into which it enters by the agency of a free acid. He considers that, in a healthy state of the system, the precipitating acid is thrown off by the skin, and he supposes that even when generated in excess, it may be diverted to the surface of the body by merely increasing the insensible perspiration. But, from whatever cause the precipitation may take place, its occurrence must be considered as a very delicate test of alimentary disturbance. By watching the occurrence and disappearance of these deposits, we are enabled to form a very just conclusion as to the efficacy of any plan of medicine or diet that may have been prescribed. I am acquainted with a gentleman who can never eat bread without discovering a change in his urine. He told me that he had entirely overcome the lithic diathesis by substituting biscuits. To those who are not acquainted with the influence which the slightest error in diet possesses over the urine, this may appear a refinement scarcely within the bounds of credibility: Dr. Prout, however, has stated a parallel case. The variety of colour, also, exhibited by the lithic sediments, is deserving of some attention, and the profession is under deep obligations to Dr.

Prout for the able manner in which he has described such modifications. He arranges them under three divisions, viz. 1. *Yellowish or nut-brown* sediment; 2. *Reddish-brown or Lateritious* sediments; and 3. *Pink* sediment. The first variety indicates a strong tendency to the lithic acid diathesis : although in some cases an opposite state of system prevails, and an alkalescent condition of the stomach and bowels may be supposed to exist, in general, the nearer such sediments approach to white, the more of the phosphates they contain. Dr. Prout says, that the second variety of sediment varies in tint from nearly white, in which state it is with difficulty distinguished from the last variety, to a deep brick-red or brown. It is to be considered as a symptom indicative of phlogistic fever, or very frequently of local inflammatory action. The third variety of sediment owes its colour principally to the *Purpurate* of *Ammonia :* its presence indicates the existence of certain chronic visceral affections, especially of the liver.

311. These observations are sufficient to impress upon the practitioner the necessity of inspecting the urine of his patient; the indications it affords are not to be received without due caution. If taken alone, they may not be worthy of any considerable degree of credit, but when viewed in conjunction with other symptoms, they will undoubtedly assist his diagnosis.

312. We come now to consider the " Particular Circumstances" of the patient under examination. His *age,* for obvious reasons, is a fact of importance. By learning the nature of his *occupation,* we shall be enabled to form some judgment with respect to the causes that may have excited his disease. The posture in which some persons are accustomed to sit, is a frequent source of affections of the stomach and bowels. Literary people and clerks from bending to the desk or table are frequently thus affected. Tailors and shoemakers are notoriously obnoxious to serious obstructions from such a cause : by the position in

which these tradesmen pass a considerable portion of the
day, the margin of their ribs is pressed upwards so as to
force the stomach against the diaphragm, and to impede
the passage through the pylorus. It is equally essential
to inquire into the *former habits and customs* of the patient;
we thus become acquainted with his dietetic irregularities,
the degree of exercise to which he has been accustomed,
and various other circumstances which may have contributed
to produce the disease under which he labours. If he has
resided in a warm climate, we shall be led to suspect the
existence of hepatic affection. The " Occasional Questions" which I have introduced, as necessary for the examination of females and children, are too obvious in their
importance to require any farther comment. With respect
to the value of " General Observations" upon the physical
character of the individual, I have only to state, that those
accustomed to medical physiognomy will derive much
information from such an inspection; although the evidence is of such a nature that it cannot be described; it
is to be learnt only by experience.

OF THE CURE OF INDIGESTION,

As it relates to Diet, Exercise, and Medicinal Treatment.

---

313. The previous habits of the patient, and the origin and seat of the disorder, are the circumstances from which the physician is to derive his indications of cure. If the disease has not extended its influence beyond the stomach and bowels, the means to be adopted will be more simple, and, at the same time, more prompt in their salutary operation, than where it has involved the functions of remote organs; but in this latter case, the symptoms are so frequently those of mere sympathy, that the practitioner has often the satisfaction of witnessing their removal by remedies that can only have acted on the primæ viæ.

314. It has been stated (257) that the stomach may fail in the performance of its duties, either from a deficiency in the secretion of its menstruum, or from a loss of power in its muscular fibres; but in either case we must refer the disease to a loss of nervous energy. Some persons, predisposed to indigestion, and who inherit the temperament most favourable to its production, would seem to have less than an ordinary ratio of nervous energy supplied to their muscular structures. In such cases, there is an unusual torpor in the bowels, even during health. An attention to this fact has frequently led me to adopt measures which might have proved less successful under other circumstances. As a general proposition it may be stated, that the secretion of gastric juice, and the muscular power of the stomach, are so intimately associated with each other, that the one cannot long be deficient without the other

partaking in the torpor; and the practitioner, who has had much experience in the treatment of dyspeptic disease, will readily concur with Dr. Philip in believing, that whatever tends to restore a healthy nervous power to the stomach, tends to form the food into that substance which is best fitted to excite the muscular fibres of this organ; and that whatever excites the natural action of these fibres, tends to relieve the nerves from their load, and, in the most favourable way, to bring into contact with their extremities the food on which, through the intervention of the gastric fluid, their powers are to be exerted.

315. The pathology of the stomach may, therefore, be greatly simplified by referring it to a defect of nervous action; and our first duty is to enquire into the causes that may have occasioned it, and which, in general, may be identified with errors of diet, affections of the mind, or irregularity of exercise.

316. The nature and influence of such remote causes have been fully discussed in the preceding pages; and by carefully appreciating their operation, the practitioner will obtain a clue for his guidance. He must lay down a system of rules for his patient, by which the remote causes of his complaints may be removed; but, in his attempts to reform bad habits, he must be careful to avoid all abrupt transitions, except in those circumstances which have no direct influence upon the vital powers of the body. I should, for instance, be very cautious how I withdrew spirituous stimulants, although I might be well satisfied that the indulgence of such potations had given origin to the disease; but I should not feel any hesitation in at once withholding every species of pastry, or other indigestible matter, without reserve. Upon the same principle, we should gradually diminish the number of meals, where they have exceeded the proper limit, adopting them with skill and caution to the fluctuating circumstances of the patient. The same observation applies to exercise: no-

thing would be more injudicious than to expose the invalid, debilitated by sedentary habits, to the effects of
sudden and protracted exercise ; nor should the person,
whose habits have been laboriously active, be abruptly restricted to an irksome state of indolence. The discipline,
in such cases, must be graduated according to the previous
habits of the patient ; to his age, strength, and the nature of
his disease. Exercise can never prove salubrious, if it be
followed by fatigue. Mr. Abernethy has prescribed to his
patients a set of rules, which I shall take the liberty of
quoting in this place, in order that I may offer such observations upon their value, as my own experience has
suggested. " *They should rise early when their powers
have been refreshed by sleep, and actively exercise themselves
in the open air till they feel a slight degree of fatigue.*"
Upon this first rule, I am disposed to make the following
comment. Although we must all agree in the advantages
of early rising, yet, in dyspeptic cases, I have frequently
known the disease greatly aggravated by the patient suddenly changing his habit, with regard to the hour of rising ;
and that if he becomes the least fatigued, before his morning repast, he remains languid and uncomfortable during
the rest of the day. A long walk before breakfast, unless
the person has been accustomed to the practice, will frequently produce a fit of indigestion. I have already observed, that it is advisable to allow an interval to pass
before we commence the meal of breakfast ; and where the
weather and circumstances will permit it, this interval
should be passed in the open air, but the body should not
suffer the least fatigue. Mr. Abernethy then proceeds to
say, " *they should rest one hour, then breakfast, and rest
three hours, in order that the energies of the constitution
should be concentrated in the work of digestion.*" It appears, then, that the patient is to rise early, to take exercise until he feels slightly fatigued, and then to rest an
hour before he is allowed to take any refreshment. This

plan might succeed very well in preserving a robust and healthy man in vigour; but where we have to deal with a person whose energies are languid, and whose feeble powers are easily exhausted, I fear that such discipline would be ill-calculated to afford assistance. It is notorious that all dyspeptic persons are especially languid in the morning, and they accordingly require a regimen the very reverse to that which Mr. Abernethy recommends. Such, at least, is the conviction of my mind. To the practice of resting three hours after breakfast there can be no objection; it is the period best adapted for intellectual business. He then recommends " *active exercise again for two hours, rest one; then taking their dinner, they should rest for three hours, exercise two, rest one, and take their third slight meal.*"

317. It is impossible to frame any general rule that shall apply to every case, but I will offer a sketch of the plan I have usually recommended: the practitioner will readily modify its application to meet the circumstances of any particular case. The dyspeptic patient should rise from his bed as soon as he wakes in the morning: for as Mr. Abernethy justly states, that " many persons upon first waking feel alert and disposed to rise, when, upon taking a second sleep, they become lethargic, can scarcely be awakened, and feel oppressed and indisposed to exertion for some time after they have risen." He should then walk, or rather saunter for some time in the open air, previous to taking his breakfast, the material of which is to be selected according to the principles already discussed (232). He is now in a condition to follow his usual avocations; but it is a circumstance of no slight importance to procure an evacuation at this period, which is easily effected by habit (79); a person who accustoms himself to the act at a certain hour of the day, will generally feel an inclination at the appointed season. The invalid should not allow his occupations, if sedentary, to engage him for more than three hours, after which exercise

on horseback, or by walking, should be uniformly taken.
I have already observed, that the state of the weather
ought not to be urged as an objection to the prosecution
of measures so essential to health.   Where the season of
the year, and the situation of the patient, will allow the
exercise, I strongly urge the advantages to be derived
from digging : the stimulus thus given to the abdominal
regions is highly salutary in dyspeptic affections.   The
hour of dinner should not be later than three o'clock
(233), and the patient should rest for an hour before
he sits down to the meal (243).   It should consist
but of few articles (227), should be carefully masti-
cated (236), and the invalid should rise from the table
at the moment he perceives that the relish given by the
appetite ceases.   The manner in which he should regulate
his potations, at and subsequent to this meal, has been
already considered (146).   With respect to the allowance
of wine, every practitioner must use his discretion, and be
guided by the former habits and present condition of his
patient (167).   It is essential that the invalid should enjoy
rest for at least two hours after dinner (106), that is to
say, he should not enter upon any occupation or diversion
that may occasion the slightest fatigue ; to a gentle walk,
or saunter in the garden, there can be no rational objection, especially at that season of the year when such a
pastime is the most inviting.   At six or seven o'clock, he
may take some diluting liquid, as tea ; after which, exercise will be highly useful, to assist the sanguification of his
previous meal : in the summer season there will be no difficulty in accomplishing this object ; and if the strength of the
patient will allow the exertion, some active game, as bowls,
will be attended with advantage.   At ten o'clock he may take
some toasted bread, or a lightly boiled egg, with a glass of
wine and water, should his previous habits render such an
indulgence necessary, and at eleven he may retire to rest.
The bed-room should be well ventilated, and its tempera-

ture should, as nearly as possible, be that of the apartment from which the patient retires. A well-stuffed mattress is to be preferred to a bed of down, and the curtains should not be so drawn as to exclude the free circulation of air. The invalid should be careful in not retiring to rest with cold feet: nothing contributes more readily to disturbed sleep, and uneasy dreams, than the unequal circulation which takes place on such occasions.

318. Such are the general rules which I should enforce for the protection of those invalids who are liable to dyspeptic attacks. There are particular features in the history of every case which will require appropriate treatment, and I shall now proceed to their consideration.

ACIDITY OF STOMACH, FLATULENCE, &c.

319. It has been a question often discussed, whether the acidity which occurs in the stomachs of dyspeptic invalids, arises from the fermentation of the food, or from a vitiated state of the gastric secretion? It appears to me that it may occasionally depend upon either of these causes. In cases of imperfect chymification, it would appear more generally to depend upon the matter generated by the food; for it is instantly relieved by a dose of carbonate of soda: but where it is symptomatic of some disease in a distant organ, as in that of the uterus, it would seem to be connected with an acid state of the gastric juice, and is not relieved by the administration of alkalies. I am not aware that this distinction has ever been established, but I am so well satisfied of its truth, that I have, in several cases, been led, from this circumstance alone, to distinguish between primary and symptomatic affections of the stomach. Unrelenting and continued cardialgia ought to lead us to suspect disease in some other organ; although I am not prepared to state that it is never the effect of a primary affection of the stomach.

320. In ordinary cases of acidity, the procuring evacuations from the bowels is the first measure to which we are to resort. We have afterwards to adopt such treatment as may prevent its recurrence. This indication is to be fulfilled by bringing the digestive organs into healthy action by a well-regulated regimen, and by such medicines as may give tone to the stomach, and increase that propulsatory action of the bowels, by which they are enabled to pass off the undigested portions of food. It is also probable that the bile may be unduly secreted in quantity or quality, for cardialgia is a common symptom of hepatic obstructions. Emetics have been recommended by some authors; but I suspect that such remedies, however quickly they may remove the present paroxysm, are calculated to favour its return. I am therefore disposed to prefer purgatives, especially as the disease is generally complicated with fœcal congestions in the colon. Five grains of the compound extract of colocynth, or of the compound camboge pill, combined with two of calomel, afford a very efficient remedy upon such an occasion. When the bowels have been thus relieved of their load, their peristaltic motion may be kept in a state of gentle excitement by the following draught, which I have found to be singularly efficacious in such cases.

R Sodæ Tartarizatæ, ℥ij.
    Sodæ Carbonatis, Ɂij.
    Aquæ Anethi, f ℥j.
    Tinct. Calumbæ, f ℨj.

Fiat haust. cum Acidi Tartarici granis quindecem in aquæ semi-fluid-uncia solutis, in impetu effervescentiæ sumendus.

321. The exhibition of alkalies and absorbent earths will remove the present evil, but it will not produce any beneficial influence in averting the cause by which it was produced. Carbonate of ammonia is, perhaps, the most efficacious of the antacids, for it neutralises a portion of the acid matter which appears to exist in a gaseous state

in the stomach, and which, on that account, eludes the action of the fixed salts. It is, moreover, calculated to relieve the debility which so frequently attends an attack of this nature. I have known very small doses of opium relieve this affection after the bowels have been thoroughly evacuated; and in cases where there is reason to refer its origin to a symptomatic affection of the stomach, nitric acid has been found useful. Diarrhœa is not an unusual attendant of this disease, in consequence of the irritation which the bowels receive from the contact of the acrid matter : small doses of magnesia, combined with a few drops of laudanum, and made into a draught with some mucilage, will generally be found to relieve the complaint.

322. We are, however, to look for permanent relief to a change in the food; all the vegetables should be withdrawn, and a diet of animal food substituted : but if such a change should excite the disgust of the patient, we must relax in our commands, for the stomach will never digest that against which the inclination rebels. The substances which are found, by experience, more particularly liable to create this disorder, are all fried articles, butter and greasy viands, pastry and crude vegetables; in short, whatever is indigestible may act as its exciting cause. Astringent wines, as port, are very apt to favour its occurrence. I have before observed, that the stomach is frequently sensible to very minute portions of astringent matter (171). Dr. Philip says, that he has known more than one instance in which the stomach was even sensible to the difference between coloured and colourless brandy. Broths of every description, but especially those made of the meat of young animals, are a fruitful source of heartburn. Veal contains a saccharine principle which is very susceptible of acetification. The medicines best calculated to invigorate the alimentary canal, are those composed of pure vegetable bitters, with the addition of some aperient salt. The infusion of quassia, in the dose of half a fluid-

ounce, with two fluid-drachms of the infusion of senna, and a drachm of tartrate of potass, warmed with some aromatic tincture, is an excellent compound in such cases. I have also found the infusion of rhubarb, quickened with a small proportion of the compound tincture of aloes, a very useful remedy.

323. Flatulence is often a very distressing disease; it sometimes is associated with acidity, but frequently is the only symptom which indicates an imperfect digestion. Whether the gas, with which the intestines are inflated, be a product of fermentation, or a secretion from their vessels, is a question which has given origin to some discussion. It may probably arise from either of these causes, although it is generally attributable to the former. In some cases, it appears to contain sulphuretted hydrogen gas, and eructations take place which are characterised by the smell of rotten eggs. Where this occurs, we may infer the existence of great alimentary disturbance; the natural affinities, by which the digestive changes are produced, appear to be subverted, and a new chain of compositions and decompositions established. The albumen would seem to be the substance from which this compound is generated; and in several cases which have fallen under my notice, relief has been obtained by confining the patient to a strictly farinaceous diet. Ordinary cases of flatus, however, are of a different nature; the air appears to be the product of fermentation, and, by avoiding such vegetables as are known to be susceptible of it, the disease has been removed. In certain states of the alimentary canal, a sense of distention may be felt, without any morbid increase in the quantity of intestinal gas; an undue sensibility or irritability of the bowels may occasion such a feeling. This fact has been well illustrated by Dr. Parry:* he observes, that " there is often consider-

* Collections from the Unpublished Medical Writings of the late Caleb Hillier Parry, 1825.

able variation in the degree of inconvenience resulting from the use of food or drinks which disagree." " Some- times," says he, " if I take acids, as considerable quantities of fruit, and immediately afterwards eight or ten scruples of kali at a dose, in saturated aqua kali carb., I feel no dis- tention of the stomach, and bring up no carbonic acid gas : several hours afterwards there is a great uneasiness in the colon, which is not relieved till a great quantity of wind passes downwards.   In this case it was absolutely neces- sary that the wind should have existed in the stomach, because an acid and an aerated kali were mixed there. But no dyspepsia, or what is called wind, was produced by it, because the stomach itself was not thrown into a spasmodic state from being over-irritable.   Afterwards, however, when the same wind passed into the colon, that bowel being in a state of morbid irritability, the uneasi- ness from the wind was produced there till the wind was expelled."   Although the terms in which this fact is ex- pressed may not be consonant with those of modern science, the fact itself, as well as the explanation of it, are of great practical value.   It is not the presence of gas in the intestinal canal, but the irritability of the intestines, which renders them impatient of the slightest stimulus of distention, that occasions the distress so common to dys- peptic invalids.   A person in robust health may, from various accidental circumstances connected with the na- ture of his food, experience an unusual intestinal disten- tion; but it will not occasion distress, for the reasons above stated.   The practice to be founded upon such observa- tions is evident: we shall obtain more advantage from calming the irritability of the bowels, than by dispelling the flatus by carminatives.   I have found small doses of the extract of hyoscyamus, combined with two grains of ipecacuan, produce relief in attacks of flatulence which have resisted the ordinary methods of cure.   Dr. Parry considers that dyspepsia consists in such a state of the

villous coat of the stomach or intestines, or both, as subjects them to be morbidly susceptible of irritation from
certain kinds of food, or certain changes of the food, which
are not perceived, or produce no uneasiness in healthy
stomachs; and that this affection of the villous coat,
throughout all its degrees, up to inflammation itself, is
apt to be followed by sympathetic or symptomatic affections of the secretory arteries or glands seated in it, and
often of the muscular coat of the alimentary canal itself.
I believe that such an affection is the general consequence,
although not the cause of dyspepsia. In the treatment,
therefore, of this complaint, we may frequently interpose
sedatives with advantage. Protracted dyspepsia not unfrequently depends upon a morbid condition of the alimentary surfaces; the mucous membrane becomes affected, and the disorder is not removed until measures
have been adopted to restore its healthy secretions. A
fretful state of the intestinal discharges is generally associated with such a disturbance, and I have found the administration of a lenient purge every morning, with small
doses of the *vinum colchici*, repeated twice a day, eminently successful in such cases. .

324. Where the dyspeptic disease is connected with
duodenal irritation, I know of no medicine more useful
than the *vinum colchici;* taking care to accompany its
exhibition with that of occasional laxatives. Purgatives
that act with violence are always followed with an aggravation of the symptoms. Dr. Yeats speaks in high terms
of commendation of the sulphate of potass : " It appears
to me," says he, " to have a more specific effect upon the
duodenum than the sulphate of magnesia. I give $\ni$j. of it
twice a day, in the infusion of quassia, and gr. iij. of the
pilula hydrargyri, with or without two grains of extract.
aloes, according to the state of the bowels. If much
feverish irritation prevails, arising, as I imagine, from
some slight inflammatory action in the duodenum, the

saline draught, in a state of effervescence, is substituted, with the sulphate of potass, for the bitter infusion, with the happiest effects, and the pil. hydrarg. is given without the aloes." This is very excellent practice : I am satisfied that nothing is more mischievous than active purgation in every stage of dyspepsia. Drastic doses of calomel, to which some practitioners resort, are calculated to increase the morbid irritability by which the disease is kept alive. In cases even of loaded bowels, it will be more prudent to excite their peristaltic action by a gentle but continued stimulant, than to irritate by active purges. Where the biliary discharges are faulty, small doses of mercury are useful; and I prefer the *hydrargyrum cum creta,* on such occasions, in doses of four grains, and combined with two or three grains of *pulvis ipecacuanhæ,* to every other form of combination.

325. Mr. Abernethy has offered some very valuable observations upon the subject of purgatives : he says that persons may be purged without having their bowels cleared of the fœcal matter which may be detained in them; we should therefore endeavour to ascertain what kind or com-bination of purgative medicines will excite a healthy action of the bowels, without teasing them, or producing discharges from the organs themselves. The best mode of proportioning the degree of excitement to the end de-signed, is to take a dose of a suitable medicine at night, but short of that which may prove irritating; if it fail sufficiently to excite the organs, a similar dose may be taken in the morning; which also failing, it may be repeated at regular intervals during the day. The prin-ciple that should govern our conduct in the administration of purgatives, may be briefly stated—*the excitement is to be repeated till the requisite action is induced,* yet no single *excitement, being such as may prove an irritant to the organ.*

326. The mischief which may be produced by too active purgation seems to have been well understood by

the ancients; but the modern practitioner has too frequently
rejected the advice which the sages of our profession have
recorded for his instruction. " He who takes a rough
purge," says Plutarch, " to relieve his body from too great
a load of food, may be compared to the Athenian, who
finding the multitude of citizens troublesome to him, contrived to drive them out by filling the city with Scythians
and wild Arabs." I do not wish to invest the Grecian
historian with the attributes of a medical oracle; but we
may be allowed to borrow from him a figurative allusion
to illustrate the importance of a precept which cannot be
too frequently or too forcibly impressed upon the mind of
the medical practitioner.

327. We may obtain the best form of a purgative from
an infusion of senna, graduated in strength according to
the circumstances of each particular case, and combined
with small doses of some neutral salt. Where accumulations may be supposed to have taken place in the colon, a
dose of the *pilula cambogiæ composita* is an effectual
remedy.

328. Where the symptoms of dyspepsia are accompanied with an evident spasmodic affection of the alimentary canal, as indicated by its inverted and convulsive
movement, the malady may be inferred to exist more particularly in the muscular structure. Dr. Parry is inclined
to regard such cases as distinct from those of dyspepsia,
and to class them under the head of *nervous irritability of
the stomach;* but they evidently constitute a link in the
same chain, and are so intimately connected with the
series that they cannot be practically separated from it.
In such cases the symptoms of flatus are prominently distressing: the air which exists in the canal, and which
should pass insensibly downwards, inviscating itself with
the food, is thus arrested in its course, producing borbo-
rigmi and eructations from the stomach. In such cases,
the medicines most likely to afford relief are aloetic stimu-

lants : I have found the *decoctum aloes compositum* a truly
valuable remedy in all affections connected with a torpid
or irregular action of the muscular coats of the intestines.
On some occasions, I have subjoined the *infusum armo-
raciæ compositum* with evident advantage.

329. The administration of the white mustard seed,
which has been lately revived with all the confidence which
attaches to a newly discovered remedy, is certainly a useful medicine in several morbid states of the intestinal
canal; but, according to my experience, it is serviceable
only in such cases as are marked by alimentary torpor.
In affections attended with muscular inirritability, or in
those associated with a diseased state of the mucous surfaces, it is unquestionably useful. I have known it to
ensure a regular alvine discharge in persons of costive
habits ; and I have also found it to correct that species of
diarrhœa which attends a diseased condition of the mucous
membrane of the intestines. These unbruised seeds were
much commended by Dr. Mead in ascites, and by Ber-
gius in intermittents, and numerous writers have extolled
their virtues in stimulating the stomach and intestines.
Dr. Cullen, however, observed that the seeds given in this
form are never broken down or dissolved in the stomach,
but pass away entire by stool; and he therefore inferred
that they were incapable of producing any beneficial
effect. This statement appears to have thrown so much
discredit upon their value, that they fell into disuse, and
they have only lately regained the confidence of the profession. I confess myself to have been amongst those
who were disposed to consider the *unbruised* seeds as
perfectly inert; but experience has taught me that such
an opinion is incorrect. The seeds consist of fecula, mucilage, an acrid volatile oil, on which their virtues depend,
and which on standing deposits a quantity of sulphur, a
bland fixed oil, which considerably obtunds the acrimony
of the former constituent, and an ammoniacal salt. The

fixed and volatile oils may be obtained by expression, and
if the mixture be submitted to the action of alcohol, the
latter will be dissolved, and be thus separated from the
former. It has been lately discovered, by some experiments conducted in France, that if the alcoholic solution
be evaporated, a solid and crystallizable substance, distinguished by acid properties, may be obtained; and as
sulphur is said to enter into its composition, it has been
termed " *sulpho-sinapic acid.*" If the whole seeds be
macerated in boiling water, we shall at first obtain an
insipid mucilage, which, like that of linseed, resides in
the skin; but if the maceration be long continued, the
water will become impregnated with matter yielding the
odour of sulphuretted hydrogen; a sufficient proof that a
portion of the volatile oil may be thus extracted; and it is
probable that this process may even proceed more rapidly
in the digestive canal. In administering them, however,
as a remedy, we should be cautious to prevent their accumulation in the bowels. A patient, to whom I lately
recommended their use, informed me that his evacuations
became extremely offensive, so that it is not improbable
that a portion of sulphuretted hydrogen may be disengaged during their passage. Their administration evidently requires caution: if any inflammatory irritation
exists, they must prove injurious: where, however, there
is a sluggish or deficient secretion of the alimentary juices,
I have no doubt respecting their utility.

330. The practitioner is well acquainted with the doctrines of Broussais: he maintains, that almost every
disease arises from an inflammatory affection of the digestive canal; and, although the absurdity of so general a
proposition must be admitted, we shall act wisely in sus-
pecting the existence of such a state of disease in protracted dyspepsia: tenderness upon pressure, and the
appearance of the discharges from the bowels, will generally announce such a condition; and lenient purges, the

application of leeches, and a low diet, will furnish the best methods of treatment.

331. The utility of bitters, in the treatment of dyspepsia, is a very questionable and often a dangerous practice. It is, however, the popular resource of those who suffer from deficient appetite; and I am satisfied that many serious evils have arisen from its indiscriminate application. Where the disease arises from a mere want of tone, and is not complicated with intestinal irritation, such medicines are, of all others, the most effectual; a truth which will be readily deduced from the observations which I have already offered upon the operation of these agents (135).

332. Blisters are of eminent service in cases of intestinal irritation, accompanied with tenderness on pressure; they will frequently also put a stop to obstinate vomiting, when other methods have failed of success.

333. The external application of heat to the region of the stomach will often allay gastric irritation that depends upon the presence of indigestible matter. The process of chymification is thus promoted by a species of contiguous sympathy that is not well understood.

334. The application of heat to the feet will be attended with the same beneficial consequences: this connexion is still less apparent, but it is a fact, no less remarkable than true, that the digestion of a person in health may be arrested by the sudden application of cold to the lower extremities.

335. The use of frictions, when applied by means of the flesh-brush to the abdominal region, deserves a distinguished place in the catalogue of dyspeptic remedies. I have usually directed its application for a few minutes, night and morning, and the most obvious benefit has arisen from it. The ancients are well known to have held friction in high estimation, not only in the cure, but for the prevention of disease. The moderns have unwisely

suffered the practice to fall into disuse. If it were necessary to illustrate the utility of friction, we have only to
adduce the well known effects which are produced on
horses by the operation of *currying ;* and which can alone
depend upon freeing the surface from the recrementious
part of the perspirable matter, and promoting a due circulation in the skin. In thus making them sleek, they
become more gay, lively, and active, and will preserve
their strength with half the quantity of food, than when it
is given to them without such assistance. In cases where
the application of cold may be considered useful, the
brush may be immersed in equal quantities of vinegar and
water.

336. With respect to the utility of wearing flannel
next the skin, some diversity of opinion has existed. Its
advantages consist in gently stimulating the surface, promoting perspiration, and conveying away the moisture as
it may be deposited. When worn only in the day it does
not appear objectionable, but is, on the contrary, salutary
to those whose skin may be supposed to require such a
stimulant ; but I agree with Dr. Beddoes in believing
that no good reason can be assigned why any one, who
is the master of a comfortable bed, should wear it during
the night. In that state of increased sensibility of the
skin which sleep induces, it is more likely to be injurious
than at any other time, by the stimulating effects of its
piles, and by the warmth it keeps collected round the
body. There is also another objection to its use, under
such circumstances : the perspirable matter, by accumulation, undergoes a chemical change, and the skin is thus,
as it were, immersed in a noxious atmosphere. For the
same reason, the flannel should be frequently changed.
I have generally preferred, in dyspeptic cases, the use of a
flannel *stomacher,* or a piece of loose flannel worn over the
stomach and bowels during the day, and which may be
thrown off at bedtime.

337. The use of cold and warm bathing offers another subject for consideration. The advantages arising from it, in the treatment of dyspepsia, are indisputable; but its application requires skill and prudence. When we consider the functions of the skin, in their relations to the digestive process, we cannot be surprised that an improvement in the state of the former should confer a corresponding benefit on the latter. The cold bath appears eminently serviceable to those who are suffering from dyspepsia, induced by the enervating modes of life peculiar to great towns, or by great mental exertion. Where, however, there exists considerable biliary disturbance, it generally does harm. It is also a matter of great consequence to ascertain the strength of the patient, and whether his vital energies are sufficient to produce that re-action, without which the cold bath must ever prove a source of mischief. This circumstance must likewise direct us in appointing an appropriate period for the operation. The robust and healthy may bathe early in the morning, or before breakfast, without the least hesitation; but the dyspeptic invalid should never venture into the water until his stomach has been stimulated by a slight meal. The period best calculated for immersion is about two hours after breakfast, which will enable him to take some previous exercise; he ought never to feel any degree of chilliness, but should be rather warm than cool, before he attempts to bathe. Dr. Currie has justly observed, " that persons ought not to wait on the edge of a bath, or of the sea, until they are perfectly cool, for if they plunge into the water in that state, a sudden and alarming chilliness may be expected, which would not have been the case had they been moderately warm when they went into the water." There exists a popular belief that, unless a person plunges head foremost, an accumulation of blood may take place in the brain. There is no truth in this observation. A sudden plunge is a violent and unnatural

exertion, and if the patient has not strong powers of re-action, it may be followed by unpleasant consequences. The shock thus given to the nervous system may, like a blow on the head, produce syncope. A case occurred at Brighton in which a person, in a state of debility, died suddenly from the shock of a shower-bath.

338. An invalid should never remain longer than two minutes in the water, and the body should be kept during the whole time under the surface. If, instead of a genial glow, chilliness, languor, and headach follow, we may conclude that the vigour of the system is not equal to create and sustain that re-action upon which the benefits of bathing must depend, and the practice should be im-mediately abandoned. It is, I think, generally advisable for invalids to bathe only on alternate days, until they find their strength so much increased as to allow them, without risk, to indulge it daily.

339. The patient generally inquires whether, before bathing in the sea, it may not be proper to prepare himself by the use of a warm bath. I generally recommend a previous immersion in the *tepid* bath, at a temperature commencing at 90° Fah., lowering five degrees each time, and terminating at 65°. Some laxative should be taken a few days before the course of bathing is commenced; but all violent purges must be cautiously avoided. I have known persons who, from a popular notion of the safety of purgation on such occasions, have taken violent doses of medicine, and been rendered extremely ill by their first immersion.

340. The warm bath is better calculated for those in-valids whose reaction is not sufficient to sustain the shock of cold water. In such cases it will augment rather than diminish their natural strength and vigour; it will regulate the functions of the skin, promote the digestive powers, and concur with other measures to re-establish their health. To ensure objects so desirable, there are several precau-

tions which it may be necessary to enumerate. As our purpose is not to induce profuse sweating, the temperature should not, on the first going into the bath, exceed 94° or 95°, but it may be gradually increased to 98°. In ascertaining its heat, we should never trust to our sensations; the thermometer is the only indication upon which we should rely. The most proper period for using the warm bath is an hour or two before dinner. If it be used during any of the ulterior stages of digestion, as in the evening, it will be liable to accelerate the circulation, and to produce disturbance. I have known persons, troubled with indigestion, to suffer considerable restlessness and irritation, by going into a warm bath just before bed-time. The patient ought not to remain immersed longer than twenty minutes; and upon coming out, he may walk in the open air, but should be cautious not to occasion fatigue. Count Rumford has published an interesting essay on the subject of warm bathing, in which he observes that " a person may gain fresh health, activity, and spirits, by bathing every day at two o'clock in the afternoon, at the temperature of 96° or 97° Fah., and remaining in the bath half an hour. He continued that plan for thirty-five days, and derived from it permanent advantage;" and he adds, " that the idea of going into bed after a warm bath, in order to prevent taking cold, is erroneous; that no alteration should be made in the clothing, and that the body, on exposure to the air, is not more susceptible of catching cold than it was before going into the bath." This coincides so perfectly with my own experience, that I feel it unnecessary to offer any farther remarks upon the subject. Count Rumford also justly reprobates the idea of any advantage being derived from temperate baths of from 55° to 60°. The animal temperature, he observes, is 98°; in those temperate baths, therefore, we lie motionless in a temperature inferior to that of our own bodies, and consequently must lose instead of

acquiring heat, or even retaining that which we possessed.

341. *Shower-baths* have been supposed to be more
efficacious, in certain diseases, than baths of less partial
application. In stating the result of my own experience
upon this subject, I have to observe, that in debilitated
habits they are not unattended with danger. I have
certainly seen that species of indigestion which would
seem to arise from, or be intimately connected with nervous
irritability, greatly alleviated by the use of such partial
baths, but I have generally recommended that the temperature of the water should be raised to 50°. Persons of a
strong habit, who have been exhausted by intellectual
exertion, are greatly resuscitated by such means.

342. *Change of air* is one of the most efficacious
methods of curing dyspeptic complaints. The chemist
has proved that the essential constituent parts of the
atmosphere are the same in all places and situations; it
has been collected in cities and in the country, on mountains and in plains, and even at the height of 7250 yards
above the level of the sea, by Gay Lussac, in his aërial
voyage in September 1805 ; but it has never been found
perceptibly different in composition. From the latest and
most accurate experiments, the proportions of oxygen and
azot are 21 and 79. It is indeed true, that various foreign
bodies may be present, such as an increased quantity of
carbonic acid, animal exhalations, smoke, &c. The quantity of aqueous vapour is also liable to constant variation.
What then renders the air of some places so much more
salubrious than that of others? or, whence arise the advantages which the invalid so constantly experiences from
change of place? The proposition itself may perhaps be
denied; and any attempt to establish an explanatory
theory upon such a subject, may be compared to the
attempt made by the Royal Society, at the command of
king Charles, to explain " why, if a vessel is filled brim-

ful of water, and a large live fish be plunged therein, that it shall nevertheless not overflow."—Is it a fact? Is one situation more salubrious than another? and do dyspeptic patients actually derive any benefit from mere change of air? I do not imagine that any physician, who has practised a few years, will require any evidence of these facts beyond that which his own experience must have supplied. It is notorious that children, who may be regarded in the light of sensible instruments, become unhealthy, if constantly confined to the air of large cities; robust and healthy persons are not so affected; but the delicate, and above all, the *dyspeptic* invalid, is notoriously injured by it. Let him retire only for a few days into the country, and the effect which is produced by the change is too apparent to admit of any question. Some have supposed that the insalubrity of the air of a large city may depend upon the greater dampness and stagnation of the air, occasioned by its numerous buildings : I am not disposed to assert that such causes may not have a share in producing the effect; but the animal effluvia, and the carbonaceous matter so abundantly floating in the atmosphere, must also be taken into consideration. How does it happen that plants wither and die in a short time after they are brought from the nursery-grounds into the more capacious streets of the metropolis? Why should iron rust with so much greater celerity in London than in the country? These observations, however, merely go to prove that the air of a city is less pure than that of the country. Is there any evidence to show that the air of different places, remote from towns, varies in its salubrity in different places, or in the same place at different times? I apprehend that most of the beneficial or evil effects of different air may be ultimately referred to its relations to moisture and dryness. That such changes are considerable and striking, under certain circumstances, have been rendered apparent by the admirable researches of Mr.

Daniel, who, by the invention of a simple and correct hygrometer, has been enabled to throw very considerable light upon this hitherto obscure subject. That the cutaneous discharge is very materially affected by the degree of moisture in the atmosphere is evident; and that the digestive organs may therefore be thus influenced, through its medium, is a corollary which no one will refuse to admit. When the air is very moist, it is a bad conductor of the perspirable matter, which, therefore, instead of being carried off in an insensible form, is condensed upon the surface; hence we appear to perspire greatly upon the slightest exercise, whereas the cuticular discharge is, at that time, absolutely less. We have all experienced the sensation of heat, and disposition to sweating, during the moist weather which so frequently occurs in this country in April and May, the wind being at the time stationary at south-west or south. On the contrary, during the prevalence of an east-wind, the most violent exercise will scarcely prove diaphoretic, and yet the quantity of cutaneous exhalation is far greater than during that state of atmosphere when the slightest exercise deluges us with perspirable matter. Dr. Schmidtmeyer says, that in Chili, notwithstanding the high temperature which would have been intolerable in Europe, and deluged the inhabitants with perspiration, so rapidly does evaporation proceed, that it might even be doubted whether, after considerable exercise, any perspiration was occasioned by it*. It is scarcely necessary to observe that the atmosphere of Chili is remarkable for its dryness. The functions of the lungs are no less influenced by the state of the atmosphere than those of the skin. The former organs are constantly giving off water, and if it be not carried off, with equal rapidity, it is reasonable to suppose that some influence will be produced upon them, beneficial or otherwise, according to the peculiar condition

---

* Travels into Chili.

of the patient, as I have endeavoured to explain in the
last edition of my Pharmacologia, under the history of
Expectorants. How is the cure of hooping-cough, by
change of air, to be explained, unless we adopt the belief
which I have endeavoured to enforce ?

343. The advantages which attend "change of air,"
in the treatment of various diseases, has been ascribed
by many physicians to the exhilarating impressions
thus produced upon the mind, and to the simultaneous
change of habits which usually takes place upon such
occasions. I am willing to admit the extensive and
powerful operation of such causes in the treatment of
diseases in general, but more particularly in those cases in
which the digestive organs constitute the source of the
derangement; for such affections are influenced by the
state of the mind to an extent to which it would be difficult to assign a limit.   It therefore follows that, in the re-
commendation of a place of resort for invalids, various
circumstances are to be taken into consideration : it is no
less important to furnish amusement for the mind, than to
provide salubrious air and wholesome food for the body.
A continual change of residence is, perhaps, better adapted
for ensuring our object, than a protracted stay in any one
place.   The genial excitement, which a succession of
novelties produces on the mind, to say nothing of the
advantages which necessarily arise from the exercise of
the body, is more likely to ensure exhilaration and cheer-
fulness, and to break down the associations which continued disease will always engender, than a monotonous
residence in a *watering place*, where, after the first few
days, the patient becomes familiarised with the objects
around him, the spell by which he is to be cured is
broken, and his mind is watching every pulsation, in order
to discover some indication of that returning health which
he so anxiously anticipates. This truth is beautifully
illustrated by an anecdote related by Sydenham, and will

go farther in establishing the importance of the principle I am desirous of enforcing, than any argument which it is in my power to adduce. This great physician having long attended a gentleman of fortune with little or no advantage, frankly avowed his inability to render him any farther service, adding, at the same time, that there was a physician of the name of Robinson, at Inverness, who had distinguished himself by the performance of many remarkable cures of the same complaint as that under which his patient laboured, and expressing a conviction that, if he applied to him, he would come back cured. This was too encouraging a proposal to be rejected : the gentleman received from Sydenham a statement of his case, with the necessary letter of introduction, and proceeded without delay to the place in question. On arriving at Inverness, and anxiously enquiring for the residence of Dr. Robinson, he found, to his utter dismay and disappointment, that there was no physician of that name in the place, nor ever had been in the memory of any person there. The gentleman returned, vowing eternal hostility against the peace of Sydenham ; and on his arrival at home, instantly expressed his indignation, in not very measured terms, at having been sent so many hundred miles for no purpose. " Well," replies Sydenham, " are you better in health ?" —" Yes ; I am now perfectly well, but no thanks to you." " No ?" says Sydenham, " but you may thank Dr. Robinson for curing you. I wished to send you a journey with some object of interest in view ; I knew it would be of service to you : in going you had Dr. Robinson and his wonderful cures in contemplation, and in returning you were equally engaged in thinking of scolding me." There was more wisdom and address in such a scheme than in that which is said to have been practised by Hippocrates, who sent his patients from Athens with no other object than to touch the walls of Megara, and then to return.

344. I have thus endeavoured to investigate the principles upon which the treatment of indigestion is to be conducted. I might have descended into fuller detail, but the art of selecting remedies, of graduating their strength, and of modifying their powers by combination, constitutes a subject to which I have directed the attention of the practitioner in a distinct work, the extensive sale of which convinces me that it must be already in the hands of every professional reader, and will render any farther observations in this place unnecessary. After all, more benefit will arise in dyspeptic diseases, from a judicious regulation of the diet and habits of the patient, than from large quantities of medicines; although I do not intend by this observation, to undervalue the importance of such agents, when directed by the skilful hand of the physician. The unhappy invalid, who seeks for relief from the nervous cordials, and stomachic mixtures of the empiric, may occasionally derive the feeling of temporary relief, from the operation of stimulants to which the regular practitioner will never resort. Let him remember that such relief, if obtained, must be at the expense of his future welfare. Such expedients have been aptly enough said to be drafts upon the constitution, payable with compound interest a few months after date.

345. I shall now recapitulate some of the more prominent doctrines which have been established in the preceding pages; a plan which will not only have the advantage of placing the subject in a simple and perspicuous point of view, but of affording the reader with a convenient index to the practical parts of the work.

RECAPITULATION.

1. The first object is to discover the origin and seat of the disease (290).

2. If it arise from a debilitated state of the stomach, in

which either the secretions are deficient or depraved, or
the musculars powers of that organ have lost their
vigour, we have first to remove, as far as we are able,
the remote causes which may have produced the disorder.
The alimentary canal must be cleared of all foul
congestions, and their future accumulation prevented,
first, by a strict adherence to a diet most likely to ensure
the digestion of the food; and, secondly, by the careful
exhibition of laxatives, which may carry off the superfluous
parts. The functions of the skin must be restored, and a
general vigour imparted to the body, by remedies which
are calculated to strengthen the nervous system.

3. If the dyspeptic disease has continued so long as
to produce an inflammatory state of the gastric membranes, we must employ antiphlogistic means for its
cure (330).

4. If the duodenum be the seat of the disorder (265),
we must carefully ensure, by appropriate diet, the complete chymification of the food, so that it shall not be
irritated by the contact of half digested food; the secretions which enter its cavity must be regulated and improved, by small doses of mercury; and colchicum may
be administered in the manner above directed (324).
Above all, the colon must be carefully preserved from
feculent accumulations.

5. If the bowels be distressed with flatus, we must
ascertain whether the feeling arises from an increased
quantity of air present in the canal, or a morbid sensibility
of the membranes, which renders the ordinary quantity of
elastic matter burthensome. In the former case the
treatment must be regulated by such measures as may
prevent fermentation (323), in the latter, the irritability
of the intestines must be appeased by sedatives.

6. If acidity prevails, we have to inquire whether it
arises from the nature of the food, or the morbid state of

the gastric juice, and regulate our measures accordingly (319).

7. Where disease exists in the bowels, and the appearance of the stools indicates a dysenteric affection, we may infer that the mucous membrane is in a state of disease.

8. The administration of tonics and aromatic stimulants will always be attended with mischief, where a phlogistic condition of the mucous membranes exists: mild aperients and light diet are to be prescribed under such circumstances.

9. Where there exists a languor in the muscular powers of the alimentary canal, and a torpor in the secreting membranes, bitters, aromatics, and other stimulants, such as mustard-seed, &c. may be safely administered.

10. The dietetic code of the dyspeptic patient may be summarily included under the following precepts :—

A. *Precepts in relation to the QUALITY of Food.*

a. Animal food is more digestible, but at the same time more stimulant and less flatulent, than vegetable diet. A dyspeptic invalid may be restricted to meat and bread with advantage, until his digestive powers have gained sufficient energy to enable him to convert vegetable matter into healthy chyle (110, 111), after which a due mixture of both species of aliment will be essential (112).

b. The wholesome quality of food depends as much, or even more, upon its mechanical condition, than upon its chemical composition (123—125) ; and as this is influenced by various circumstances under our own control, we may render food, naturally indigestible, of easy digestion (126—128). The digestibility of any species of aliment, as well as its nutritive qualities, are influenced by the different modes of cookery (129—134). The addition of condiments is also capable of producing the same effects (135—142). The practitioner will be enabled to direct that species of food, which is best calculated to fulfil the indications of the case, by an attentive perusal of thóse remarks which are introduced in the body of this work (189—227). And he will also find ample directions for his guidance in the selection of liquids for drink (143—186).

B. *Precepts in relation to the* QUANTITY *of Food.*

a. This must, in every case, be regulated by the feelings of the patient : let him eat slowly, masticate thoroughly, and, on the first feeling of satiety, dismiss his plate, and he will not have occasion for any artificial standard of weight and measure. But he must, in such a case, restrict himself to one dish ; an indulgence in variety provokes an artificial appetite which he may not readily distinguish from that natural feeling which is the only true indication (236—241).

C. *Precepts, with regard to the* PERIODS *best adapted for meals, and on the Intervals which should elapse between each.*

I have, upon every occasion, endeavoured to impress upon the practitioner the high importance of these considerations. In every situation of life, we too frequently pass, unheeded, objects of real importance, in an over-anxiety to pursue others of more apparent but of far less intrinsic value ; so is it with the dyspeptic invalid in search of health : What shall I eat ? Is this, or that species of food digestible ? are the constant queries which he addresses to his physician. He will religiously abstain from

whatever medical opinion, or even popular prejudice
has decried as unwholesome; and yet the period
at which he takes his meal is a matter of comparative indifference with him : although he will refuse
to taste a dish that contains an atom of vinegar
with as much pertinacity as if it held arsenic in
solution, he will allow the most trifling engage-
ment to postpone his dinner for an hour.   So important and serious an error do I consider such
irregularities, that I have frequently said to a patient
labouring under indigestion, " *I will wave all my
objections to the quality and quantity of your food,
if I were sure that such a sacrifice of opinion would
ensure regularity in the periods of your meals.*"

a. The principal solid meal should be taken in the
middle of the day (233).

b. Four hours after which a liquid meal should be
indulged in (234).

c. The digestion of one meal should be always completed before fresh labour is imposed upon the stomach
(98).

d. The intervals at which food is to be taken must be
regulated by the digestive powers of the individual,
and the rapidity with which they are performed
(233).

e. The patient should never take his meal in a state of
fatigue (243).

f. Exercise should always be taken three or four hours
after dinner (105, 245).

On the Diet best adapted for Persons labour-ing under Tabes Mesenterica.

We know nothing of the operation of the mesenteric
glands, nor of the part they perform in the scheme of

digestion; but we are assured, by experience, that when they become diseased, emaciation and atrophy follow. The dietetic plan which I am about to propose in such cases, was neither suggested, nor am I aware that it can be successfully supported, by physiological theory; although, if it were my object to adduce an hypothesis, I think I might be able to give it the air of plausibility. My conviction of the utility of the treatment, however, rests exclusively upon the basis of experience. I have uniformly found a vegetable diet injurious in such cases, while one entirely composed of animal matter has proved beneficial; but in order to ensure such a result, the meals should be scanty, and in quantity short of what the appetite may require; the intervals, also, between the repasts should be lengthened. In this way are the unwilling absorbents induced to perform their duty with greater promptitude and activity; but it is a practice which, from the extreme anxiety of friends and relatives, the feelings of craving and hunger expressed by the patient, and the mistaken but universal prejudice respecting diet, it is always painful to propose, and generally difficult to enforce: where, however, circumstances have given me a full and unreserved control, the advantage of the plan has been most decisive. In affections of this kind, the stomach rarely loses its powers; and it is less an object to provide easily digestible, than highly nutritive food. I have a patient of this description, who has derived much advantage from a diet composed principally of animal fat; and I have frequently noticed a sort of instinctive desire for rich and concentrated nourishment, which has not produced the ill effects which it undoubtedly would have occasioned in a simple dyspeptic disease.

OF THE DIET OF PULMONARY INVALIDS.

In tubercular affections of the lungs, it has been often disputed whether the low diet, so universally prescribed in such cases, is that which is best calculated to arrest the progress of the disease. From my residence at Penzance, and from the various cases which have fallen under my care, in consequence of having there practised, I may, without the risk of incurring the charge of presumption, assert that few physicians have possessed greater opportunities of experience in this complaint than myself. The conclusions to which this has led me may be expressed in a very few words. Where there exists, in the earlier stages, great lassitude, coldness of the extremities, a quick but weak pulse, a tightness across the chest, as if it were confined by cords, but unaccompanied with acute pain in the side, a strictly vegetable diet is injurious. I have in such cases prescribed a regimen similar to that which I have above proposed for the cure of mesenteric affections; and I have certainly found it to be useful. To assert that I have cured an organic disease in the lungs would be more than foolish; but I have certainly arrested its progress in some cases, and I have restored others to perfect health, who had been gradually declining under a different treatment. Where a permanent cure has been effected, the presumption is, that the lungs were never actually deranged in structure; but the symptoms were of a nature to have justified such a conclusion. The medicine upon which I place the greatest reliance in such cases, is the extract of hemlock; and were I to express the extent of my own confidence in its powers, I might, perhaps, fall into the dangerous error, against which I have so strongly protested in my Pharmacologia—that of bestowing such extravagant praise upon a remedy as to detract from its reputation. I shall, therefore, only observe, that this remedy tranquillizes the irritation of the lungs to a greater degree than any other medicine with which I am acquainted; but in order to ensure so desirable an effect, it must be given in much larger doses than those in which it is usually adminis- tered. I usually commence with a dose of five grains three times a day, which I gradually increase to Əj, or even more: it will generally produce a slight giddiness, nausea, and a tremor of the body; a peculiar heavy sen- sation is also experienced about the eyes, and a tightness across the forehead; and the bowels frequently become relaxed: unless some of these sensations are produced, I consider that the remedy has not had a *fair trial.* The following is the formula for the preparation of the mixture which I have found to be so highly serviceable. If I am required to explain the *modus operandi* of each ingredient, I might, perhaps, fail in inspiring that confidence in its utility, to which I am convinced it is entitled. The practitioner must therefore rest satisfied with the results of experience, and accept facts in the place of theory.

    ℞ Extract. Conii, et
        Extract. Hyoscyami, āā Əij.
        Mucilaginis Acaciæ, fℨij.
   Tere simul, et adde
        Liquoris Ammoniæ Acetatis, f℥j.
        Aquæ puræ, f℥ivss.
        Vini Ipecacuanhæ, fℨj.
        Syrupi Rhæados, fℨij.
   Fiat mistura, de quâ sumantur cochlearia duo ampla ter quo-
      tidie.

I have now fulfilled the objects which I proposed to myself in the composition of the present Work. I have attempted to establish the principles upon which the di- gestibility and nutritive powers of different aliments de- pend; and I have endeavoured to point out the circumstances which may render any species of food indigestible and noxious. I have shewn the causes upon which dyspepsia depends, and enumerated the remedies which may be applied for its cure. It only remains for me to relate a few Cases in illustration of the views I have offered, and in confirmation of the utility of that medicinal and dietetic treatment which has been developed in the preceding pages.

CASES

CASE I.

A. B., a gentleman of rank and fortune, of the age of twenty-four years, had suffered for several months with occasional headach in the evening, which, at first, was generally relieved by a cup of strong coffee, and it therefore excited little or no attention. The pain, however, became more severe, and returned at shorter intervals; it sometimes attacked him during the morning, and was accompanied with sickness, by which a quantity of strong acid was ejected from the stomach, and the paroxysm was thus terminated. His person was strong and athletic, his countenance florid, and he underwent considerable exercise during the pursuit of the field amusements to which he was devoted : his appetite was therefore considerable, and the quantity of food which he was in the daily habit of taking, exceeded that which is generally sufficient for the most robust. He had never been in the habit of restricting his diet, because he had hitherto never felt any inconvenience from its excess. In the use of wine, however, he was temperate. The first professional communication which I received from him was in April 1824; he had then for some weeks been suffering from headach and sickness, and distressing symptoms of acidity. I shall quote that part of his letter in which he describes the treatment he had received. " My medical attendant ordered me aloës and blue pill, and a potion made of gentian, bark, cascarilla, and liquor potassæ. I found the prescriptions, word for word, in your Pharmacologia. I cannot, however, say much for them, although the draught certainly does me some little good: he also ordered me lime-water, which is worth all the other put together: as for magnesia, I might as well eat powdered glass. What do you recommend next? I am regularly feeding on mutton, beef, &c., to the utter disgrace of vegetable diet." From this period he gradually grew worse; his attacks of headach increased in severity and frequency, and were rarely relieved until a great quantity of bile and intensely acid matter were thrown off the stomach: he grew rather thinner, but was by no means emaciated. I ordered him doses of carbonate of ammonia an hour after his dinner, and desired him to confine himself to an animal diet. He was well purged, and the action of the bowels kept up by small portions of a neutral salt. The stools were always natural in appearance. He now found the slightest deviation from the prescribed diet to produce a headach; and when he prognosticated its approach from the presence of acid eructations, he was frequently enabled to avert it by a dose of ginger and carbonate of soda, which I had also prescribed for him. He says, " I have found it necessary to take your prescription once or twice a day, which has averted many a vile headach, as I always take it if I feel any symptom of the generation of acid, such as heartburn, or an acid taste in my mouth. Having thus converted ' my stew-pan, vat, mill, &c.' into an apothecary's shop, I am much better than I have been, and have been nearly free from headach for the last fortnight, until yesterday, when I was in dock all day, and shall be so to-morrow. There is still, however, remaining to plague me, a sort of languor and laziness which perhaps Dr. C.'s bitter prescription is intended to obviate, though it scarcely has such an effect. I wish the shooting season had arrived." I have introduced the relation of his feelings in his own words, because they will serve to convey a good idea of their nature and intensity, as well as of that hilarity and natural flow of spirits which constantly accompanied the progress of the disease of this highly-gifted and amiable young man. In November I received from him a letter, of which the following is an abstract: " I find that the perpetual recurrence of my old headaches leaves me nothing for it but to turn them into a subject of amusement. I have been reading some speculations about muriatic acid in the human stomach, and would like very much to know what acid is in mine; and I wish you would put me in the way of testing it, for I can obtain any quantity. If it is a vegetable acid, how does it get into giblet soup or salt beef, or fresh butter, *cum multis aliis*? if it is an animal acid, I know of none except the phosphoric, and I have no idea of making a match-box out of my viscera, so I vote at once it is not that; if it is a vegetable acid, how comes it that I may eat a dozen *ripe* peaches, and be none the worse for them? but woe to me if I eat a buttered muffin; *ergo*, I infer that it is not wholly the acetic acid; and if not, what else can make *sweet* tea, or any thing like ale, beer, or porter, perfect poison to me? As for an animal acid, there is no poison for me like strong broth, or soup; *ergo*, there must be some villany in that. I was told, the other day, that baked meat would disagree with me, and I find this to be the case. Now, for the muriatic acid, which I strongly suspect to be the one under which I suffer, for the action on my teeth, when I am sick, is too sharp for any thing less pungent; I find that if I eat salt meat, an acid is immediately formed in my stomach, and yet I can take any quantity of salt with my meat, without being the worse for it: how can this happen? I am so often almost frantic with these headaches, that I am quite willing to devote myself to any experiment which you may choose to institute. The next curious, and to me unaccountable fact is, that if I eat *any thing*, even a mutton chop, between breakfast and dinner, I am sure to suffer from it, and that severely. About a week ago I went to Dublin, to transact some important business, and, lo, when the day came, my head felt as if it were nailed to my pillow. They sent for Mr. Crampton, the surgeon general, who greatly approves of the carbonate of soda and ginger, and added to it five grains of rhubarb. This very day I have taken, at three times, thirty grains of the soda, which gives a very temporary relief. I am particular in my diet, and take no drink but water; still, in spite of these precautions, I have a very bad headach once a week, and a moderate one or two besides. It is very odd that I never had two of my severe headaches on two successive days; that they never make me look the least pale or yellow. Their progress is exactly similar: I am at first heavy and dull, then a headach comes; then I *feel* sick, then I *am* sick; the produce of the operation is very acid, or very bitter; then I get better, and go to sleep, but in a quarter of an hour I wake worse, and so on, every half hour until about four in the morning, when I gradually get better, and invariably wake quite well."

By a steady perseverance in the plan of diet and medicines prescribed for him, he found considerable alleviation, until April 1825, when he complained of having a return of his old headaches, with their usual severity; but he had relaxed in the strictness of his diet; and he adds: " I think, by more care in future, I shall be able to keep them in check; but I ought to state that I now suffer from a sense of weight and oppression, chiefly after meals." On the 18th of May he had a most violent attack, owing to having eaten a mince pie, and his subsequent letters complain of a listlessness and want of energy, which rendered him incapable of the slightest exertion. I expressed a wish to see him, and he arrived from Ireland on the first of June; the journey had been of service to him, and I found him much thinner, but

better than I had expected. His numerous friends in
London, anxious to pay that respect which his talents
and urbanity so justly commanded, poured in their in-
vitations, so that to expect obedience to any plan of regimen was not to be calculated upon. He left London,
and proceeded to Leamington, where he unfortunately, by
the explosion of his fowling-piece, lacerated his little finger,
and was compelled to suffer its amputation. His health
declined under this operation; he lost flesh, experienced
increased headaches, and was so ill as to induce his friends
to call in the aid of a popular practitioner in that neigh-
bourhood, under whose superintendance he took drastic
doses of scammony, not only without relief, but with an
evident aggravation of the symptoms. He became thinner,
and more than proportionally reduced in strength; so
much so, that he found himself incapable of horse exercise: he suffered severely from constant nausea and oppression. In this state he continued, until his bowels,
for the first time since the commencement of the disease,
exhibited signs of torpor. " From a daily pill of camboge,
scammony, aloes, and colocynth," says he, " I was obliged
to increase the dose to four, and at last to discontinue
them as entirely inefficient; and medicine having become
as necessary to me as food, my medical attendant in Ireland has contrived a more active combination, which I
take daily, but I fear that I shall be obliged either to increase its dose, or supersede it by one still more powerful,
as I find that this is even losing its effect." His bowels
at length became so torpid, that the most powerful
drastics failed in their operation; his strength was daily
declining; scarcely a day passed without headach and sickness: he suffered, during the night, from most violent
cramps in his legs. In the middle of December I received
a letter from him, which was nearly illegible; and he states
that he can scarcely see his hand, not from dizziness, but
from an indistinctness of vision, which continues without

any amendment during the day. His vision at length became so imperfect, that he could no longer correspond with me: I then urged the necessity of his once more coming to town; a proposal which he eagerly embraced; but such was his weakness, and so severe his sickness, vomiting without any cessation for forty-eight hours, that he was many days on the road. His face, hands, body, and legs, swelled to a considerable degree, and he experienced great difficulty in breathing. As soon as he arrived in town, I immediately proposed a consultation. His bowels had not been moved for ten days, and every medicine given for that object had failed in its effects: this circumstance, connected with the fact of his deficient vision, which now rendered him incapable of recognising his friends, or even of distinguishing the window-frames, induced me to suspect that all the symptoms of this unfortunate case were to be referred to some disease in the brain. Sir H. Halford, Dr. Maton, and Dr. Warren, met me in consultation. The first great indication to be fulfilled was the evacuation of the bowels; he had already, by my direction, taken ten drops of the oil of the *Croton Tiglium* without effect. He was now directed to take twenty grains of calomel, with five grains of scammony; and a dose of the infusion of senna, with jalap and a neutral salt, every hour, until an evacuation was procured. After some hours the bowels answered, and a perfectly healthy and figured motion was obtained. The vomiting was appeased by effervescing draughts; and a trial of the hydrocyanic acid was proposed. He was cupped, and blistered on the back of the head; but his vision grew daily more obscure; his headach was relieved, but he constantly experienced a sense of weight and uneasiness in the region of his stomach; his pulse was regular, but hard, and rarely less than a hundred beats in a minute. In this distressing state he remained for ten days; when I was suddenly called to him in the middle

of the night, in consequence of a violent dyspnœa which
had seized him. I found him in a state of apparent suffocation, and immediately requested the attendance of
Mr. Keate, in order that some blood might be abstracted
from the arm. He lost sixteen ounces, but no relief was
afforded by the operation. Dr. Maton saw him shortly
afterwards with me : hæmorrhage had taken place from
the lungs, and he died at two o'clock, after the failure of
the methods usually adopted in such an exigency. What
was the nature of his disease? I confess that I had long
considered the brain as its seat; and I explained the
dyspnœa from a deficient supply of nervous energy, his
symptoms bearing a striking analogy to those which were
produced by a division of the eighth pair of nerves. The
result, however, of the dissection will throw some light
upon this obscure and interesting case. Upon inspecting
the abdominal viscera, not the slightest trace of disease
could be discovered; the stomach was larger, and the
diameter of the intestines smaller than usual, but there
was no other appearance worthy of notice. On opening
the thorax, the lungs appeared so gorged with blood, as
almost to resemble the spleen in texture; they were
emphysematous in several places. The heart was apparently healthy in external appearance, but of a large size ;
upon making an opening into the right auricle and ventricle, these cavities were morbidly dilated, so as to constitute what has been termed *passive aneurism :* their
parietes were not thickened. The left ventricle was also
unusually large : the valves were in a healthy condition,
Upon opening the head, the structure of the brain and
its membranes were found in a perfectly healthy state, but
without the usual presence of blood. The substance of
the brain itself was perfectly blanched, and, upon cutting
into it, the usual spots of blood were not produced. This
organ, therefore, although not injured in structure, must
have been unfitted for the performance of its functions

from a deficiency of blood; in consequence, probably, of the feeble action of the heart. The history of this extraordinary case will admit of much physiological speculation. That the heart was the primary seat of* the disease, appears to be the most probable conjecture; the loss of vision must have arisen from a deficient circulation through the brain; and to this also we are to attribute the obstinate state of the bowels. The derangements of the stomach may be referred to its sympathetic relations to the stomach. The gorged state of the lungs may be accounted for, either by the imperfect action of the heart, or by the deficiency of nervous energy; for a similar appearance is observed in cases of narcotic poisoning, where the death of the animal takes place from the destruction of the powers of the brain. I have lately met with a case of diseased heart, in which the patient complained of a similar imperfection in his vision; and he died in consequence of pulmonary hæmorrhage. I had no opportunity of examining the body.

CASE II.

C. D., a gentleman resident in the country, and far advanced in life, was seized with a violent pain in the gastric region at two o'clock in the morning: he arose from his bed, walked for some time about his room; and at length, the pain having left him, he again retired to rest, and awoke in the morning perfectly well. This paroxysm returned every morning, at about the same hour, for several weeks: his medical attendant administered large doses of calomel, from a conviction that the disease

---

* I have learnt, since his death, that the pulsations of his heart frequently produced a considerable noise in bed, but he was himself unconscious of it, and never experienced the least unpleasant feeling in the chest; nor did the pulse, or any other symptom, indicate disease in that organ.

arose from some hardened fæces in the colon; but this treatment aggravated the complaint. He afterwards gave him five grains of *pil. hydrargyri* every night, and a dose of neutral salt in the morning; but the disease continued to harrass him with more or less violence every successive morning. Under these circumstances, he proceeded to London for advice, and placed himself under the care of a physician of celebrity, who decided at once that the liver was the seat of the disease. The patient was accordingly subjected to a course of mercury; his gums were affected, but still no alleviation of the pain was experienced. It was several weeks after this event that I first saw him, and the effects of the mercury had subsided. My first object was to inquire into the state of his digestive functions, with a view to ascertain the length of time which his organs required for the completion of their operations. It appeared that his digestion was unusually slow, and that one meal in the day was amply sufficient to satisfy his wants. He dined at six o'clock, and I therefore thought it probable, that at the period when he was usually awoke out of his sleep by pain, the food might be undergoing its ulterior changes in the duodenum. I carefully examined the seat of this complaint; there was evidently a puffiness in the region of the duodenum, and, by pressure, he experienced a slight pain, which extended into the lumbar region. I directed him to change his dinner hour from six to three o'clock, and I laid down for his guidance such a plan of diet and exercise as would be best calculated to ensure a perfect digestion. I also prescribed the following mixture : —

> R Mist. Camphoræ, f ℥vss.
>   Vini Colchici, f℈ij.
>   Magnesiæ Carbonatis, ℈j.
>   Spir. Juniper, Co. f℈ij.
> Fiat mistura, de qua sumantur cochlearia duo ampla, mane nocteque.

I saw him after the interval of a week : he informed me that he had entirely lost the pain, and that his bowels had been gently relaxed by the medicine. His tongue, which was previously furred, had become clean, and no pain was now produced on pressure. He called upon me several times, and left London perfectly cured.

CASE III.

E. F., a young man, twenty-six years of age, and a clerk in one of the public offices, applied to me under the following circumstances. Previous to the attack of which he complained, he had enjoyed very good health, although his bowels were constitutionally sluggish, and he had been in the habit of taking, occasionally, a purgative pill to excite them into action. He was attacked with a sense of oppression in the region of the stomach, accompanied with an uneasiness in his head, and great depression of spirits. His skin was harsh and dry, his tongue furred on the back part, and his appetite was greatly impaired. He awoke in the morning with a parched mouth, and a feeling of lassitude which he had never before experienced. His urine deposited large quantities of lithic acid : he was unable to give me any satisfactory account of the appearance of his alvine evacuations ; I however desired that measures might be taken in order to obtain the necessary information. I directed him to take a pill composed of five grains of the compound extract of colocynth, and two grains of calomel, at night, and a draught of senna, with sulphate of magnesia, in the morning. It produced four copious evacuations of highly offensive matter, of a greenish hue, and mixed with a quantity of undigested matter, like soft soap. He experienced a feeling of relief, but still his uncomfortable sensations were not removed. After an interval of three days the dose was repeated ; the evacuations were more healthy in appearance, but his symptoms were rather aggravated by the medicine. His head felt heavy, and his ideas were confused. His pulse was perfectly natural. I directed him to take three grains of the *pil. hydrargyri*, with two grains of the powder of ipecacuan, every night, and to take each morning a draught composed of three fluid-drachms of the infusion of senna, six fluid-drachms of mint-water, and a drachm of tartrate of potass. His diet and habits he had told me were perfectly regular, and that his occupation would not allow him to alter the hour at which he took his dinner. At this period I lost sight of him for several weeks; his friends had persuaded him to apply to some other practitioner, who, as I afterwards learnt, had directed a very proper plan of medicine for his cure; but he daily became worse, lost flesh, and suffered much from uneasiness in his head : he had, at his own desire, been cupped, but the operation afforded no relief. On his return to me, I found him labouring under all the symptoms of protracted dyspepsia, and the greatest depression of spirits. I told him that nothing short of a complete revolution in his habits would cure him ; that it was in vain to expect relief from medicine, unless its administration was associated with a strict adherence to such a plan of regimen as I should propose. He reluctantly consented to obey my injunctions. I learnt from him that his usual habit was to breakfast at nine o'clock, to proceed to his office at ten, where he continued till five o'clock, after which he walked for two hours, and dined at seven, or sometimes later. I was satisfied that this plan had gradually debilitated his digestive organs, and rendered them inadequate to the healthy performance of their functions. His mind had been exhausted by the duties of the morning, and his body by the fatigue consequent upon exercise at so unfavourable a period. I desired him to dine at three o'clock, to take some tea at six, and to walk for an hour afterwards : the only medicine which was directed for him was a draught of a saline aperient every morning. He continued this plan of diet for six weeks, and was perfectly restored to health.

CASE IV.

G. H., the active partner in an extensive firm in the west end of the town, applied to me for advice, in order that he might be relieved from a severe attack of heartburn and flatulence, which invariably assailed him every evening. He informed me that he had tried every species of food for his dinner; sometimes restricting himself entirely to animal food, and at others to a vegetable diet; that he had taken water, and drank wine, but that no perceptible difference was experienced. His usual hour for retiring to rest was eleven o'clock; but, although fatigued by the labours of the day, he was unable to close his eyes before two or three o'clock in the morning. I told him that I suspected the error was not in the quantity or quality of his food, but in the periods at which it was taken, and requested that I might be informed as to his general habits in this respect. He told me, that such was the nature of the business in which he was engaged, that it was impossible for him to leave the counting-house before six o'clock, and that he could not therefore dine before seven; but, as he commenced business at an early hour, he was compelled to take a luncheon at three or four o'clock. I immediately discovered the origin of his complaint; and told him, that he must either abandon his meat luncheon, or convert it into a regular dinner: for the simple fact was this, that the digestive organs were thus rendered unable to dispose of the second meal, since the stomach was called into action before the food, of which the luncheon consisted, was converted into chyle. I ordered him no medicine, but he called upon me after the interval of a fortnight, and informed me that he had entirely lost all his unpleasant symptoms, having made an arrangement which enabled him to dine at his house of business at five o'clock, and to return home to tea at eight.

CASE V.

K. L., a gentleman of forty-five years of age, who had long indulged in the luxuries of the table, and sacrificed liberally to Bacchus, was attacked, about six months before I saw him, with severe symptoms of dyspepsia, loss of appetite, pain and distention after eating, depression of spirits, loss of strength, restless nights, and various other symptoms, which it is unnecessary to enumerate, were sufficient to mark the nature and intensity of his complaint. He had been under the care of different practitioners; but the treatment suggested for his relief had been unsuccessful. When I first saw him, there was considerable tenderness in the epigastric region, his tongue was furred, his bowels extremely irregular, being sometimes relaxed, and at other times obstinately costive; he had occasionally passed stools loaded with mucous matter, and tinged with blood. His pulse was quick and small. He complained particularly of attacks of fever, which occasionally assailed him in the evening; they were preceded by nausea, and a slight shiver; he then became extremely hot, and his head throbbed: this feeling continued for three or four hours, and left him extremely languid and dejected. He was unable to account for these paroxysms: sometimes he fancied that they might have been induced by exposure to cold, at other times he referred them to some indigestible food which he had taken. I frankly told him, that, unless he would strictly conform to the plan of diet and medicine that I should propose, I considered him in a hazardous situation. I directed him to be cupped on the epigastric region, and to take two grains of ipecacuan, with five grains of the extract of hyoscyamus, every night. I prescribed a laxative draught, composed of tartrate of soda, with a small quantity of manna, in a vehicle of mint-water, to be taken twice a day. His diet was directed to consist of the most digestible and least stimulant species of animal food, to be taken but once in the twenty-four hours, at about three o'clock. I advised him to take thin gruel with dry toast for his breakfast, and to use a tepid shower-bath on alternate mornings. I saw him again in the following week. There was less tenderness in the epigastrium, his bowels had been slightly relaxed, and he thought himself rather better, but there was no material improvement in his general health. I impressed upon him the importance of persevering in the plan, and allowed him to take two glasses of claret, diluted with an equal bulk of water. I did not see him again until after the expiration of a fortnight. He was then evidently improved, and told me that he felt confident that the plan upon which he was proceeding was the right one. He had already experienced less uneasiness after his dinner, and slept better. I found his pulse fuller, and at the same time slower. I now prescribed for him doses of the *vinum colchici*, with magnesia, in mint-water, and desired that the pills of ipecacuan and hyoscyamus might be continued. At this time he went into the country, and I lost sight of him for two months; but he returned very much better: his tongue was now clean, his bowels regularly acting twice a day, but he had still no appetite; I therefore ventured to prescribe an infusion of calumba, adding to each five ounces an ounce of the infusion of senna, and two drachms of tartrate of soda. He continued this medicine regularly twice a day, for three weeks, and is at this time so far recovered, as to be able to take two mutton chops for dinner, without experiencing any unpleasant feelings after the meal. I consider this simple plan to have succeeded in correcting the alimentary secretions, and imparting tone to the digestive organs; and I have introduced the relation of the case, merely to shew that the most aggravated case of dyspepsia may be cured by a strict adherence to a judicious diet, with scarcely any other medical remedies than such as are calculated to keep up a gently increased action of the bowels.

I could adduce many similar cases; but my object is to avoid prolixity. I trust that, in the preceding pages, I have succeeded in demonstrating the great importance of a well-regulated diet, and in establishing the principles upon which the digestibility and indigestibility of various aliments depend.

THE END.

LONDON:
PRINTED BY J. MOYES, BOUVERIE STREET.

Printed in the United States
By Bookmasters